Proceedings of the II Hague Workshop on Short-Term Dynamic Psychotherapy,
Ziekenhuis Leyenburg, November 12–13, 1980

II Hague Workshop on Short-Term Dynamic Psychotherapy

Editors
J.A. Hartzuiker and *J.H. van Birgelen,* The Hague

2 figures, 1 table, 1981

KARGER

S. Karger · Basel · München · Paris · London · New York · Sydney

Drug Dosage

The authors and the publisher have exerted every effort to ensure that drug selection and dosage set forth in this text are in accord with current recommendations and practice at the time of publication. However, in view of ongoing research, changes in government regulations, and the constant flow of information relating to drug therapy and drug reactions, the reader is urged to check the package insert for each drug for any change in indications and dosage and for added warnings and precautions. This is particularly important when the recommended agent is a new and/or infrequently employed drug.

S. Karger AG, P.O. Box, CH–4009 Basel (Switzerland)
Printed in Switzerland by Thür AG Offsetdruck, Pratteln
ISBN 3–8055–3449–3

Advances in Cardiology, Vol. 24

1st International Congress on
Cardiac Rehabilitation, Hamburg 1977

Cardiac Rehabilitation

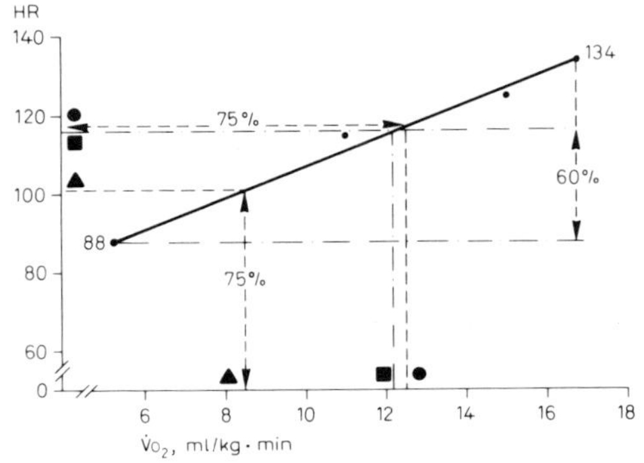

Comparison of different methods for calculating training HR from maximal or symptom-limited exercise.

Editors
K. König, Waldkirch
H. Denolin, Brussels

VI + 202 p., 58 fig.,
21 tab., 1978
SFr. 98.– / DM 117.– /
approx. US $ 58.75
ISBN 3–8055–2827–2

This volume records papers presented at the first international congress on cardiac rehabilitation, where experts convened to discuss methods and principles of therapy. Information is provided with the goal of reducing the physiological, psychological, and social consequences of myocardial infarction and, if possible, lessening the risk of recurrences and increasing the life span.
With an emphasis on practical factors, papers consider the validity of physical training programs and critically evaluate the prescription of sports and professional activities. Other sections cover psychological methods of approach and methods of secondary prevention. Practical aspects are also discussed in papers dealing with the economic and social results of rehabilitation as well as the organization of treatment centers. Through such contributions, the volume provides a critical view of the fundamental aspects of rehabilitation. A subject index is included.

Contents

Evaluation of Cardiovascular Functions
Therapeutic Aspects
Psychological Aspects
Results and Future

S. Karger
Basel · München
Paris · London
New York · Sydney

Contents

Editorial
In Cauda Venenum
Birgelen, J.H., van 217
STDP, for Better and Worse
Hartzuiker, J.A. 218

Short-Term Psychotherapy, a Major Development for Patients and Psychotherapy
Van Londen, J. 221
Short-Term Dynamic Psychotherapy: Its History, Its Impact and Its Future
Sifneos, P.E. 224
Training in Short-Term Psychotherapy. Research Can Be Superb Clinical Training
Heiberg, A.N. 230
Short-Term Psychotherapy and Hypnosis
Frankl, F.H. 236
Psychoanalysis and Brief Psychotherapy: Some New Considerations on the Psychotherapeutic Process
Gilliéron, E. 244
Short-Term Psychotherapy for the Borderline Personality Disorder
Leibovich, M.A. 257
Short-Term Dynamic Psychotherapy: Progress, Problems, Perspectives
Pierloot, R. 265

Book Review 271
Author Index 272
Contents Vol. 35 ..... after 273

Acknowledgment

The editors want to express their gratitude to those who cooperated in making the II Hague Workshop on Short-Term Dynamic Psychotherapy a meaningful experience.

With special regards to the authors, Hoffmann-La Roche B.V., Mijdrecht, Ministry of Health and Environment, Leidschendam, Municipal Hospital Leyenburg, The Hague, and National Fund for Mental Health, Utrecht.

Editorial

Psychother. Psychosom. *35:* 217 (1981)

In Cauda Venenum

J.H. van Birgelen

Ziekenhuis Leyenburg, The Hague, The Netherlands

T.S. Eliot has written: 'Genuine poetry can communicate before it is understood.' Unfortunately, this is not true for scientific matters to be printed in an international journal. To improve understanding is the editor's job.

Until now, I never had any experience in editorial work. Now I can state that it is a labour of love and hate. It has been amazing to see how some authors are able to write without bringing about any editorial problems, and others can make such problems even without writing. There must be in the latter activity a hidden or unconscious message to whom it may concern. So far my hatred.

It has been written on one of these pages that intervention in STDP ought to be considered as a creative activity. In my opinion and recent experience there is no such thing as creativity without preceding destruction. Sometimes I had to intervene in the preliminary text in a destructive way; but – believe it or not – the ultimate motive was to be constructive and corrective in a non-emotional sense. To give one example: most speakers at the II Hague Workshop, who are the present authors, will surely miss their persistent numbering of paragraphs and sentences. I have considered that inclination as a fear of losing something, to be protected by endless, somewhat obsessive repetitive counting. I'm sure that the page numbering by the publishers will be a sufficient and satisfactory guarantee that nothing of the author's papers will be lost.

It has been said that psychoanalysis is in its essence one way of looking at people and their problems. Probably writing is one way for people to present their problems. As such this editorial review has to be considered. I hope it conceals neither the relief nor the satisfaction of having been able to contribute something to the II Hague Workshop on STDP.

Editorial

Psychother. Psychosom. *35:* 218–220 (19981)

STDP, for Better and Worse

J.A. Hartzuiker

Ziekenhuis Leyenburg, The Hague, The Netherlands

After spending time organizing the II Hague Workshop on Short-Term Dynamic Psychotherapy (STDP), I am convinced that all my defenses will break down in a short while. The morning after the last farewell I woke up feeling bad due to the end of the official duties and to the prevailing feeling of loss. Having experienced the 'giving up – given up' reactions, I only could develop an 'operational way of thinking'.

Only by occupying myself with concrete reality, shall I be able to survive, since feelings, let alone emotions experienced, are not permitted.

My denial will not persist, however, because soon I shall realize that workshops and symposia on STDP provoke – next to questions on research and outcome – a major change in participants.

With a somewhat fanatic grimace, I tried to convince myself and my department that all the troubles had been for a good cause.

It is not an exaggeration to state that the Dutch have a longing for great enterprises; take, for example, the building of dikes and the reclaiming of the Zuider-Zee in a fight against the sea. So my feeling is a well-known and familiar phenomenon in these damp nether lands. It should be said, nevertheless, that my personal commitment to such an endeavour made me worry: as in any addictive dependence only the input of new discussions about STDP could take away my restlessness and somatic discomfort.

Things got worse for me after four personal confrontations with STDP during the past year. If there had been only one guru of STDP, it would have been relatively easy to demonstrate to the psychiatric world, that I recently discovered realistic, common sense reasons for hope.

It became evident, however, that there are several spiritual leaders of STDP. I survived this multiplicity by using a splitting process. Never before have I experienced the triangular situation in such an anxiety-provoking way. I got confused, for example, with all kinds of TPP links. Hidden conflicts suddenly emerged and were clarified. Discussions about 'ideation' intrigued me and I realized that I had 'to look into all that'. Finally, however, I was encouraged by the thought that our cause was indeed a great one.

To be concrete: I wanted psychotherapy in the Netherlands to change. Motivated, aware of psychological issues, capable of verbalizing feelings and experiences and having at least five enduring relationships, I felt able to promote STDP and to resist the traditional trends in psychotherapy.

I was happy to realize a beloved, maybe also disturbing fantasy: 'To concentrate nine short-term therapists in one workshop of my own.'

In organizing such a workshop even for narcissistic reasons I was a *recidivist,* for good reasons. *Pierre Schneider* used the word 'récidivé' in his introduction to the 'IIe Symposium International de langue française sur les psychothérapies analytiques brèves' [Psychol. Med. *3:* 543, 1980]. 20 years ago *Schneider* taught me the possibilities and the significance of STDP. He stressed both its advantages and its limitations. He emphasized that interventions and interpretations are creative performances, and that STDP always has an aspect of innovation both for patients and therapists. After my confrontation with short-term psychotherapists I came to realize once more that this was correct.

The more I have seen and understood and the more I have experienced – in a defenseless way – demonstrations of practical solutions to practical problems, the more I am convinced that STDP, its frame of reference being different from its application, is a real therapy for real people.

A Hague daily, on the occasion of the II Hague Workshop, put it as follows: 'It has to be a good therapy, for short-term therapy has the interest of the health authorities.'

The impact of STDP and its potential are presented by the following statement of a patient during an interview:

'You merely get oil on your wheels. I was fascinated by the experience that one can work on oneself, unconsciously. I realize my way of functioning in certain situations. Perhaps one is afraid of one's own feelings and then one ascribes them to others'. Furthermore, he added: 'I did not experience this therapy as if one person is demanding and the other is performing. I realized that I thought «if it has to come from him, it can come from anybody». *I* have to do it. That insight came to me when I was menaced by feelings of total dependence.' 'Now I have the feeling that I can recognize specific situations and that I can do something about them. I think I have the tools to do it.'

I agree with *Schneider* that a psychotherapeutic technique is more useful if the therapist has the possibilities of setting limits, and when his interventions create a real new potential for the patient. Making use – in a proper way – of common sense, insight, feelings and relations, STDP is not a pipe dream, but a real and powerful psychotherapy.

Psychother. Psychosom. *35:* 221–223 (1981)

Short-Term Psychotherapy, a Major Development for Patients and Psychotherapy[1]

J. Van Londen

Ministerie van Volksgezondheid en Milieuhygiene, Leidschendam, The Netherlands

I wish to make some brief remarks on the opening of the II Hague Workshop on Short-Term Dynamic Psychotherapy (STDP). My main point is that STDP has a major and beneficial impact not only on the patients but also on psychotherapy itself. For the patients, this therapy opens important new horizons for resolution of their psychological difficulties. To psychotherapy, the short-term time limit offers a golden opportunity for investigation of the patient selection, the therapeutic process and the outcome.

In further elaborating these points, I shall not consider the specific form of short-term psychotherapy that you are going to hear about during the next 2 days by the main speakers, who, by the way, are all pioneers in this field, and in reference to this I want to congratulate the organizers of this workshop for succeeding in bringing all these speakers to the Netherlands.

I do want to emphasize a number of technical characteristics which, according to the literature, are common in most forms of short-term psychotherapy. They can be divided into three broad theoretical categories: psychoanalytic, behavioural and crisis.

In addition, I want to enumerate certain technical aspects, which are worth paying attention to. These are: rapid, early assessment of appropriate candidates; limitation of therapeutic goals; focusing on actual therapeutic content; activity of the therapist; flexibility of the therapist; promptness of intervention; ventilation and catharsis; development of a working relationship so as to set up a therapeutic alliance, and resolution of dynamic conflicts.

[1] Opening address on occasion of the II Hague Workshop on Short-Term Dynamic Psychotherapy, November 12–13, 1980.

It should also be stressed that this kind of psychotherapy demands a great deal from the patient as well as from the psychotherapist. Patients with good ego strengths who have an acute onset of symptoms, are generally considered to be better candidates for short-term therapy than more severely disturbed individuals. It is of interest, however, that recent clinical and research findings demonstrate that short-term therapeutic interventions at times can help even the more severely disturbed patients.

It is usually assumed that the therapist should be a highly experienced professional who keeps the therapeutic goals clearly in mind and does not pursue irrelevant subjects. Since, at the start of the treatment, the problems of the patient must be quickly determined, it is obvious that experience is required. Individuals who qualify for short-term psychotherapy do present a wide range of difficulties, so the therapist should be capable of mobilising feelings of stimulating insight and of enhancing problem solving.

It is assumed that a therapist of limited theoretical orientation cannot become a good short-term psychotherapist. The development of this treatment is important to the patient, because it helps filling the gaps of his psychological functioning.

Generally speaking, psychotherapeutic contacts invariably seem to be of brief duration. A recent American survey of 979,000 patients established an average of 4.7 patient-therapist contacts. Unfortunately, such data are unavailable in the Netherlands.

Other studies show that a large percentage of patients stop their treatment after the first six to eight sessions. Interpretation of this phenomenon is not easy. It has probably to do with the premature disappointment in the contact with the therapist which was planned to be of long duration. It is also possible that many patients seek aid with an expectation that treatment will be fast and short. The latter is said to apply particularly to individuals of a lower social-economic class or of a lower educational background. But surely, it is clear that an increasing number of individuals come seeking help for a specific solution to well-defined problems, and not expecting a general personality overhaul.

In addition, it can be stated that short-term psychotherapy is an alternate for longer treatment. Although *Luborsky* et al. conclude from their survey that no significant differences are found in the outcome evaluation between time-limited and time-unlimited therapy, the Handbook of Psychotherapy and Behaviour Change emphasises that short-term therapy is not only more efficient in terms of professional time invested, but also in measurable terms it appears to be as effective. These considerations are, therefore, stimulating some therapists to apply short-term therapy as a rule and not to consider longer treatment before trying short-term therapy at first.

As a third consideration, I call your attention to the possibility of the application of short-term therapy on a broader scale. This may save considerable treatment time on an overall basis and increase the range of treatment possibilities. The editors of the above-mentioned Handbook already assumed that brief therapies would be more widely utilized in the future, if governmental health plans and private insurance companies would cover the costs of psychiatric treatments.

Research in short-term psychotherapy can also facilitate the study of the psychotherapeutic process and contribute to the evaluation of the therapeutic outcome. It has been shown, for example, that short-term psychotherapy is a valuable analogue to long therapy. It offers possibilities for the study of the effectiveness of specific interventions on specific problems. Research in brief psychotherapy may help us understand how psychotherapy can be effective.

Furthermore, the setting of realistic treatment goals between therapist and patient, gives, in my opinion, a possibility to confirm whether the chosen treatment is going to fulfil these goals or not.

In summary, the relationship between the insight, which has been achieved even on a cognitive and realistic basis, and the emotional experience, indicates that short-term psychotherapy is of major advantage to the patients in general and to the efficacy of psychotherapy in particular. Still, more work must be done on the selection criteria (indicating which patients qualify for the various forms of short-term psychotherapy). More research is also needed to specify which factors in therapeutic interventions have the most favourable effect on the therapeutic outcome.

Finally, there are good opportunities for improving the training in psychotherapy for our young therapists. Thus, any training plan devised for psychotherapists, must always include experience in short-term psychotherapy.

For us in the Netherlands it is important to modify our training model and to re-examine it completely, so that we can reflect on where in the health care system short-term psychotherapy can be best performed under the most favourable conditions.

I have tried to be brief, just as it is your aim in your short psychotherapy. I hope that the next 2 days will be inspiring to all of you and that they will give you a realistic basis for developing short-term psychotherapy in this country. With this wish I am pleased to declare your workshop open.

Psychother. and Psychosom. *35:* 224–229 (1981)

Short-Term Dynamic Psychotherapy: Its History, Its Impact and Its Future

Peter E. Sifneos

Harvard Medical School, and Beth Israel Hospital, Boston, Mass., USA

Key Words. Short-term dynamic psychotherapy · History · Research · Future · Impact

Abstract. Short-term dynamic psychotherapy is successful for the healthier patient, but also for the individual with severe and chronic problems. The author surveys the history of brief intervention since *Freud.* Despite favorable outcomes, there has been a lack of interest for short-term dynamic therapy. Analysts, emphasizing on long-term analysis, failed to distinguish between developing theory and treatment. Since the mid-fifties interest for short-term techniques has increased. Research is resulting in criteria for selection and outcome. Utilized are active techniques, as transference interpretation, in dealing with specified foci. Successful outcome is obtained in oedipal problems, grief reactions, obsessive compulsive illnesses, multiple phobias and some boderline disorders. In future, research is necessary on differentiation between patients, on comparison between treatment methods, and on technical factors, next to education and training.

That short-term dynamic psychotherapy has become popular during the 1970s is an undisputable fact. One, however, must raise the question as to why there has been such a sudden popularity about an area of psychiatric treatment which is not new and which nevertheless has its roots in the early part of the twentieth century. Is it only because third party payers have to give less money to those whom they insure? If so, the value of this kind of psychotherapy will soon be questioned, its scientific effect will be doubted, and its fashionable fame will be diminished.

In this paper I shall try to demonstrate why short-term dynamic psychotherapy has become one of the most successful therapeutic interventions not only for the healthier patient populations with circumscribed neurotic difficulties, but also for individuals suffering from severe, incapacitating and chronic psychological problems.

There are innumerable examples recently and in the distant past of very brief types of intervention which produced dramatically successful results. *Freud,* for example, was able to help cure some patients, few of which were famous individuals such as *Gustav Mahler* and *Bruno Walter* whom he saw four or five times and whose problems he was able to help resolve. Furthermore, in some of his published case reports one is struck by the fact that the early psychoanalyses had only lasted for very few months. What may be surprising, however, is that 20 years later efforts were being made to shorten psychoanalysis, because it had become unusually long-term, and at times it was going on interminably. Such efforts by *Ferenczi* and *Rank,* however, failed to have an impact on other analysts who continued to treat their patients intensely, seeing them several times a week over a period of many years, and making no effort to state for whom their treatment produced beneficial results, and for whom it did not.

The lack, therefore, of specification of criteria for selection of appropriate candidates to receive psychoanalysis or long-term psychoanalytic psychotherapy, created enormous problems. The waiting list, for example, became a standard in all psychiatric clinics and many an analyst or analytically-oriented therapist had patients who had to wait for long periods of time before they could start their treatment. All in all, many patients remained untreated and became progressively more frustrated. It is well known, however, that these untreated psychological difficulties did not disappear but were expressed in various ways, such as, for example, in the form of somatic complaints, increased alcohol intake, poor work performance and decreased productivity, as well as in more subtle interpersonal conflicts which nevertheless produced, in their relationships, innumerable problems and at times gave rise to catastrophic complications.

During the 1940s, *Alexander* and *French* obtained very meaningful results with a shorter term psychoanalytically-oriented therapy, whose effect produced 'a corrective emotional experience' on the patient and which in turn was instrumental in overcoming his difficulties. Despite these favorable outcomes, however, little attention was paid to it by the majority of the analysts who kept emphasizing the universal application of long-term psychoanalytic psychotherapy, which was thought should be offered to all mentally ill patients suffering from all sorts of conditions including psychotic and psychosomatic disorders. The tragic error which they made was the failure to distinguish between psychoanalytic theoretical principles and psychoanalysis as a treatment modality, the first being vital for understanding the human mind, while the latter being a psychiatric treatment of limited value.

By the mid-1950s work done simultaneously at the Tavistock Clinic in London by *Malan* and at Massachusetts General Hospital by *Sifneos* without knowledge by either group of the others existence demonstrated that well-motivated patients with circumscribed neurotic conflicts could be helped by psychodynamic interventions of brief duration. Criteria for selection of patients and for successful outcome were formulated. Active techniques using, for example, the parent-transference link interpretations, and dealing with specified dynamic foci such as unresolved oedipal problems or grief reactions, were utilized extensively. Finally, results of these brief dynamic psychotherapies were presented during various International Conferences and publications started appearing in great numbers pointing to successful outcome in long-term follow-up studies.

More systematic research investigation using experimental and control patients were initiated in the 1960s and were greatly expanded by the extensive use of videotapes in the 1970s. These audiovisual presentations demonstrated extensively not only the whole process of the brief dynamic therapy, but also the patients' behavioral patterns before and after their treatment and a long time after its termination.

At the same time at the Montreal General Hospital *Davanloo* had also been working on short-term dynamic psychotherapy, and in 1975, 1976 and 1977 he organized International Congresses on this subject using audiovisual presentations extensively. The enthusiastic response to these demonstrations was possibly due to the fact that the effectiveness of short-term psychotherapy had been demonstrated not on an anecdotal basis but rather on solid evidence available to the scrutiny of scientific observation. For the first time not only could research in psychotherapy be performed, but also a basis for future investigation could be prepared meticulously.

As the 1970s came to an end, short-term dynamic psychotherapy had aroused, as mentioned already, great interest in Europe and in North America, and demands for training in this field increased enormously. Unfortunately, these educational needs could not be met fully. In addition, intensive efforts were being made to enlarge the scope of brief dynamic psychotherapy by attempting to utilize these techniques with sicker patients. It was discovered, for example, by *Davanloo,* that some individuals suffering from chronic obsessive compulsive illnesses and multiple phobias responded favorably to these brief dynamic interventions. Encouraged by these findings, and by the work of *Leibovich* with certain kinds of borderline patients who seemed to do quite well over a relatively short-term period, we have tried at the Beth Israel Hospital to specify criteria for selection for these patients. Although the greatest difficulty in these individuals probably has to do with their inability to establish a give and take type of relationship due to their difficulties in separation and individuation, nevertheless, we were able to discover two elements in their character structure which seemed to play an important role in the success of their treatment.

The first criterion had to do with their *motivation to change* and willingness to overcome their problems. This criterion, which plays a crucial role for the selection of healthier neurotic patients, seems also to be significant in these borderline individuals who, despite their chaotic functioning, do try over and over to face the vicissitudes of their psychological conflicts, and occasionally with the help of their therapist are capable of solving them.

We have used seven subcriteria to assess *motivation for change* in selecting patients to receive short-term anxiety-provoking psychotherapy. These are well known by now since they have been described in the literature, but nevertheless, I shall list them briefly in this report for those who are not acquainted with them. They are the following: (1) A recognition that the symptoms are psychological in nature. (2) Honesty in reporting about themselves. (3) A willingness to participate actively in the treatment. (4) Introspection and curiosity about themselves. (5) Willingness to change. (6) Realistic expectations about the results of the treatment. (7) Willingness to make a reasonable and tangible sacrifice.

The second criterion involved the discovery that some borderline patients were *able to function effectively in one specific area of their lives.* They showed, for example, that they could perform effectively at work or academically. A young woman whose academic performance was superior, presented all the other traits of a chaotic borderline functioning in her relationship with people. Despite these difficulties the therapist was able to help this patient utilize her ability to work successfully at college and try to use this talent in other areas of her life. When the relationship between patient and therapist had been solidified and a therapeutic alliance could be developed, despite some very stormy sessions during the early part of the treatment, the psychotherapy proceeded uneventfully and ended successfully.

In retrospect it was thought that the therapist was able to create an atmosphere within the therapy which was conducive to the establishment of what *Alexander* had called a *a corrective emotional experience* when he first wrote about brief psychoanalytic psychotherapy in 1946. It was the patient's motivation to change, however, and willingness to overcome her difficulties, despite overwhelming odds, which helped her achieve a successful outcome in the final analysis.

Similar results were obtained with other borderline patients who did show an ability to function well in a specific area of their lives. It is hoped that as we go along investigating the positive response of these seriously disturbed individuals who do well in psychotherapy over a relatively short period of time, we may be able to specify additional criteria for selection which will help us differentiate these patients from other borderline individuals who may require much longer psychotherapeutic interventions.

The questions which we must pose at this point have to do with the future. What is it that we should be doing during the 1980s as far as brief dynamic psychotherapy is concerned?

First and foremost we should pursue the systematic differentiation of patients who are good candidates to receive a variety of short-term psychotherapies and who respond well to them. Each one of these therapies should be based on a clear-cut description of specified criteria for selection. Each one should clearly describe the technical requirements which are being used, and each one's outcome findings should be investigated extensively with long-term follow-up studies. It would be a serious mistake, for example, to compare patients who are good candidates to receive short-term anxiety provoking psychotherapy (STAPP) whose therapeutic focus involves a solution of an unresolved oedipal problem, with patients who are good candidates for brief dynamic psychotherapy as practiced at the Tavistock Clinic and whose therapeutic focus involves the resolution of morbid grief reactions. In the area of research we should try to develop control studies so as to demonstrate convincingly that our short-term dynamic therapies are indeed superior for a selected group of individuals to other forms of psychiatric treatments such as behavior modification or pharmacotherapy for this same group of patients.

More work should be done on identifying additional and possibly more subtle specific technical factors which are utilized during the therapeutic interventions and which may play a significant role in bringing about a successful outcome. It is time that the prevailing myth that only nonspecific factors are of any importance in psychotherapy is put to rest once and for all.

In the area of education the demand for additional training in short-term dynamic therapies will continue to increase during the 1980s. This presents a serious challenge to us. At present, only in a few centers is short-term psychotherapy taught systematically under individual supervision primarily to trainees who are working there. Some of these centers which are located in Europe, are: The Tavistock Clinic in London, and the Clinics of the University of Louvain, Liège, Hamburg, Lausanne, and Oslo.

In North America they can be found at: The Montreal General Hospital, the Beth Israel and University Hospitals in Boston, the Beth Israel and South Beach Hospitals in New York, and the Langley Porter Clinic in San Francisco.

The increased use of continuous education seminars and workshops for those interested to learn how to utilize short-term dynamic psychotherapy techniques will help increase the number of available therapists. It is hoped, however, that the national governments should establish fellowships for training and should provide financial support for education and research in this area, which up to the present time has been totally neglected. For, after all, these are the very governments which will have to subsidize more and more the ever increasing expenses of medical care.

Finally, it is imperative that some sort of international organization be set up to coordinate the training of short-term psychotherapists and by organizing large symposia or smaller workshops to present, particularly with extensive use of audiovisual aids such as videotapes, the developments of research and clinical work in this field. The possibilitiy that such an organization might be established here in The Hague, in the heart of Europe, with such excellent facilities, and so much support from governmental agencies, is a very exciting prospect. It will make all of us look enthusiastically to a bright future for short-term dynamic psychotherapy for the rest of the twentieth century.

Prof. Peter E. Sifneos, MD, Associate Director, Department of Psychiatry, Beth Israel Hospital, Boston, Mass. (USA)

Psychother. Psychosom. *35:* 230–235 (1981)

Training in Short-Term Psychotherapy

Research Can Be Superb Clinical Training

Astrid N. Heiberg

Institute of Psychiatry, Oslo University, Oslo, Norway

Key Words. Short-term psychotherapy · Research · Training

Abstract. Experiences in Norway since about 1970, are described in combined research and training on short-term dynamic psychotherapy. Research methodology and results are not discussed. Initiated by the Norwegian Research Council for Science and the Humanities, *Sifneos* was invited as research leader and supervisor in a study of STAPP carried out by a selection of highly motivated doctors participating in patient selection, training in short-term dynamic principles, activities, and research. The initial patient interview took place in front of the research group. Therapeutic activities were registrated on audiotapes and presented to the group members, each one being supervisor or supervisee alternately. The project has promoted knowledge and skill in short-term therapy and interest in research and the author stresses the fruitful interaction of both.

Introduction

There is no contradiction and not necessarily any competition between psychiatric training and conducting clinical research. On the contrary, the systematic collection of information and the comparison and scrutinizing of data can be a superb way of methodological clinical training. This paper will describe the experiences we have in Norway in research and training in short-term dynamic psychotherapy.

How to Start from Scratch

The tradition of conducting systematic dynamic psychotherapy is relatively short in Norway. It was not until the 1960s that a real interest for a systematic approach was taken in psychoanalytically-oriented psychotherapies, and not only in traditional psychoanalysis. The 1960s were characterized by a generalized optimism in psychiatry, partly due to the introduction of psychoactive drugs and partly to the increased awareness that psychoanalytical principles might be useful as a general approach in psychiatric treatment. Optimism and critical evaluation are not always closely connected. The need to critically evaluate the results of psychotherapeutic interventions was felt more in some academic circles than in the psychiatric institutions. In the beginning of the 1970s there was no on-going research in psychotherapy in Norway. The decision to initiate such research was made in the Norwegian Research Council for Science and the Humanities. The Council decided in 1970 that they would give a grant for a foreign guest professor to stay 1 year in Norway to create an interest for research in psychotherapy. We had to invite a foreign professor since we had no tradition of our own. The questions were: Which professor? What kind of psychotherapy? What method must be chosen?

Choosing Research Leader

Prof. *Peter E. Sifneos* of the Harvard Medical School, Boston, Mass. was invited. The main reason to choose *Sifneos* was the impression he had made upon Norwegian psychiatrists on his previous visits to Norway, where he had given seminars presenting his well-defined selection criteria, technical interventions and outcome data for patients treated by short-term anxiety-provoking psychotherapy. This had created a strong interest among practising Norwegian psychiatrists.

The Research Council particularly favored his work on comparing treated and untreated patients, a scientific endeavor that ought to be repeated by other researchers. *Sifneos* accepted the invitation on the condition that he could have the grant turned into a travel grant by which he could visit and supervise a research group over a lengthy period.

Choosing Topic of Research

The second question was which form of psychotherapy we should concentrate upon. There were two main issues. On the one hand we wanted to work with the psychotherapies that might prove useful for the majority of our patients, who were supposed to be rather disturbed and probably more in need of supportive integrative psychotherapies. On the other hand *Sifneos* could present us with a clearly-defined psychotherapy with a view to selection of patients, the technical aspects of activities, as well as assessment of outcome. This is a rare possibility in psychotherapy, still very few therapeutic varieties have this theoretical framework. Since we did have some realistic ideas that research in psychotherapy might be difficult, we chose to take the way that seemed to give the lesser resistance – that is to take part in a study of short-term anxiety-provoking psychotherapy.

Finding the Researchers

The third question was: who should be the researchers? The idea of doing research had come from the Research Council, but who would do the job? Our initial ideas were that this highly complicated matter could only be pursued by the most experienced psychiatrists at the University Clinic. But motivation is a decisive factor, not only in the patients but also in the therapists. It was therefore decided that we should start with a pilot project. We should challenge the assumption that the majority of our patients did not fulfill the selection criteria for short-term anxiety-provoking psychotherapy. To test this, we undertook a study where a half-year population of all the patients admitted to the hospital, were assessed, according to the selection criteria for short-term anxiety-provoking psychotherapy. That meant that every doctor in the hospital had to take part in the evaluation of the patients. For that half-year period, which covered most of spring 1972, altogether 26 doctors took part in the study. Of these, 12 doctors wanted to commit themselves to learn how to treat patients in short-term anxiety-provoking psychotherapy, and these 12 doctors formed two groups, each consisting of 6 persons.

Group Supervision

The next task was to select patients according to the criteria that had been spelled out for a short-term anxiety-provoking psychotherapy, and to treat these patients with a focusing technique using every transference situation to make interpretations on the connections between past experiences, present problems and the apparent patient-therapist transference link. Also, we should describe the outcome of the therapies and make appropriate work on the follow-up. The problems we had in selecting patients, our methodological considerations and the preliminary results, are not the topic of this presentation. I shall rather describe the impact that the magic word – research – had upon our clinical work in the groups.

Because we were doing research, we had to make sure that we agreed upon the selection criteria for the patients, and we had to make sure that we were actually conducting focused dynamically oriented short-term psychotherapy. Therefore, we had to document and demonstrate our activities and the therapeutic process. The patients were interviewed in front of other colleagues. In the beginning we used one-way screens, but the patients resented to be cut off from the rest of the audience, they wanted to see to whom they were revealing their secrets, and we, the therapists, were confronted with the fact that our own anxiety of exposing ourselves to colleagues was more prominent than the patients'. One of the reasons for this anxiety might be our previous experiences in supervisory settings during specialist training, were criticism and comments about the therapists' interviewing style were painful. In the case with the short-term patients, however, the main point was to scrutinize the evidence we had from the interviews that the patients fulfilled certain criteria. Therefore, the criticism that inevitably did occur was more that we lacked certain information, than about the therapists' general style and behavior. This made the discussion more objective and less anxiety-provoking for the therapists, and therefore more genuine and real. The natural benefit was also that the therapists exposed more of their personal style, therefore opened up for real learning both on the part of the interviewer and on the other group members. Since the discussions were taking place within a certain frame of reference, the interviewer had a much greater sense of control in the situation than he normally would feel. And when he had a sense of having control, he did not have to keep it.

In the supervision of the therapies, we also had to demonstrate to the other members of the group what we were doing, and the therapists reported consecutively to the groups. It was a great advantage that most of the members of the group had seen the patient at the group interview. This increased the interest in the patient, and possibly made the supervisory process more accurate.

A problem was whether we should use auditapes or videotapes. For several reasons we chose audiotapes, and this gave a much more vivid picture of what was taking place in the therapy than just written reports. Written reports were also used since we could not play a full therapy session, so we combined demonstrations and reports.

The groups had no formal leaders. Even if there were substantial discrepancies between some of the participants as to formal psychotherapeutic education, nobody was expert in conducting short-term focused psychotherapies, so the sense of equality was quite realistic. This also enhanced the process of openness in the group, since everybody alternated between being a supervisee or a supervisor.

During the first 2 years, there were some changes in the groups: people left and came. Eventually, one single group of 6 therapists formed out of the original group of 12. The 6 of us have had a steady group going since 1974. An important feature in the success we have in maintaining our group has been the general consensus that we should give top priority to the group work.

Modelling

Another important aspect of our training was learning by modelling from the guest professor. For the first years we were using the majority of our time when he visited us in attending his interviews with patients. The motivation for learning was high since we knew that we were going to try this on our own until his next visit. Another point of interest is that we did not have trouble in getting patients who were willing to be interviewed in English. This was a smaller obstacle than we had thought it would be.

Ripple Effect

A phenomenon which the group has experienced is that the group activities not only give training in clinical work, but also in general research methodology. Most of us have changed jobs several times during these years, but the unmistakable trend has been that we have gradually gone into research positions. This research does not necessarily limit itself to short-term psychotherapies. Other major research fields have been psychosomatic problems in patients with muscular tensions, crisis interventions at industrial disaster, symptomatology in borderline patients, and suicide rates in a cancer population. Only 2 of the members are presently preferentially doing research in short-term psychotherapy, one describing the therapeutic process in more details. In this work we are now getting valuable help from another foreigner, Prof. *David H. Malan* from the Tavistock Clinic in London.

Another aspect has been the generative effect of interest in short-term psychotherapy. 3 of the members of the group have been supervisors in three groups who are doing systematic short-term psychotherapies.

Summary and Conclusion

The most important factor in promoting training and research in psychotherapy has been the guest professor. He brought practical knowledge, served as a teaching model, and has been an enthusiastic and charismatic uniting person for the group.

Another prerequisite for the work has been the high motivation on the part of all members of the group to learn these specific skills. For some the main motivation was for learning a clinical method, for others the main motivation was to do research. But in the long run, the research aspect has gained a much greater influence than anticipated. This process can be carried on by new groups working in the same basic model.

In summary, the initiative that was taken 10 years ago has been very fruitful in promoting a climate in Norway both for advanced knowledge and skill in conducting clinical work in short-term psychotherapies, and in promoting an interest in research, and these two phenomena interact.

Prof. Astrid N. Heiberg, MD, Institute of Psychiatry, University of Oslo, Vinderen, Oslo (Norway)

Psychother. Psychosom. *35:* 236–243 (1981)

Short-Term Psychotherapy and Hypnosis

Fred H. Frankel

Harvard Medical School, and Beth Israel Hospital, Boston, Mass., USA

Key Words. Short-term psychotherapy · Hypnosis · Phobias

Abstract. Phobic patients have been shown to be, on average, more hypnotizable than others. The essence of the phobic experience is not unlike that of the event of hypnosis, and the phobic experience might be a spontaneously occurring panic-filled trance-like or dissociative experience. This dissociation is viewed as a maladaptive mechanism of defense against anxiety, sadness or rage. In addition to enabling the patient to develop a psychodynamic understanding of the symptoms, the therapist uses hypnosis and self-hypnosis to help the patient learn more about his dissociative capacity, to become familiar with the mechanism, and to learn to control it. This offers him a way to master the shift in his functioning.

Hypnosis

Hypnosis, since its *discovery* more than two centuries ago by *Franz Anton Mesmer* [1774] has been explained by many theories, several of which appear to hold a germ of truth; but in a large number of instances they are influenced by the unbridled imagination of the theorist. There are few, if any, who still support *Mesmer's* Fluid Theory involving *animal magnetism,* but the mysticism and the *magic* engendered by his actions and his theories have tended to linger in the minds of many, often to discredit the effects of hypnosis as some form of legerdemain. More recent theories have invoked the forces of the unconscious, the placebo and other factors. Clearly we cannot dwell here on all the arguments, but we can focus on a brief event of hypnosis and on a few highly relevant findings that have emerged from the laboratory investigation of the phenomenon.

A very brief version of but one of many typical hypnotic events might run as follows. The patient is asked to close his eyes, to feel himself slow down and relax, to become totally calm all through, and then to imagine himself drifting, floating or gliding. He is then told that in this state he can be keenly aware of the sensations in his limbs and in his body, and that if he concentrates on the feelings in his fingers, hand and forearm, he might just begin to experience movement sensations and then light feelings in that limb. He is encouraged to experience the feelings and then given the suggestion that the forearm and hand will become so light that the limb will rise and lift from the arm-rest to move into an upright position. When this is achieved he is told that he will not be able to place the forearm back on the arm-rest of the chair and keep it there comfortably until the therapist imforms him that he can. He might even be challenged to try to replace it before then. With his arm levitated the therapist will discuss one or more topics with the patient, or help him to understand different aspects of his behavior. When the planned treatment procedure has been concluded the therapist directs the patient to open his eyes, to be wide awake, and to return his forearm to the arm-rest; at that point he is also told that all the usual sensations and control will return to his limb and that he will continue to feel relaxed and comfortable and experience a feeling of well being.

Traditional use of hypnosis has focused either on helping the patient recall his past emotional experiences (thereby aiding the anamnesis or facilitating an abreactive experience) or on providing suggestions to help in the diminution or removal of symptoms. Both of these strategies can be applied in hypnosis while the patient sits passively, with attention focused on the therapist's comments. A variety of explanations or suggestions can, of course, be presented at that time.

At this juncture, it might be helpful to focus on what we believe hypnosis is, and on what we have learned about it. Stripped of the important facilitating factors of the hypnotic situation such as the trusting and somewhat archaic relationship with the therapist, the motivation and the preparedness to experience the event, and the relaxation and positive expectations [*Shor,* 1962], the essential aspect of the experience itself appears to be an altered state of awareness, or an altered perception; altered cognition and altered memory may similarly be part of the event [*Orne,* 1959]. This alteration of perception on a consenting basis is well demonstrated by the light feeling in the levitated hand and forearm; it is equally well exemplified by having the patient experience a numb feeling in his mandible if he is to undergo dental work, or a sense of great calm and self-mastery to succeed a feeling of anxiety. It is also in evidence when a subject is encouraged to experience a heat wave, or a blizzard, and perceives himself and his environment accordingly. It is thus useful to view hypnosis as a great adventure in imagination, and we know from well-conducted studies that persons who are highly hypnotizable do indeed have the capacity to be intensely involved or absorbed in imaginative fantasy [*Hilgard,* 1970; *Tellegen and Atkinson,* 1974].

There are clear and purposeful implications in this last statement that people vary in their capacity to experience hypnosis. This aspect of hypnosis has long been recognized by clinicians. Laboratory investigators, through the development of standardized hypnotizability rating scales, have confirmed the clinical observation and enlarged upon it [*Hilgard,* 1965]. We know from a survey of many thousands of subjects that hypnosis is not experienced in similar fashion by all. Hypnotizability is not universally distributed, and the capacity to experience it seems to be remarkably stable [*Diamond,* 1974]. This means that poor subjects are not likely to become good ones, and that good subjects, provided the circumstances are appropriate, will generally respond well. In addition, we know that a good response has little or nothing to do with the sex of the patient or the operator, nor with the patient's level of education. We have also learned that personality measures such as the Rorschach, the Thematic Apperception Test and others do not correlate with hypnotizability in the volunteer student populations that have been studied [*Hilgard,* 1965].

Phobic Behavior and Theories

Prior to the early 19th century, phobic disorders had not been differentiated from morbid fears and other morbid conditions. Their recognition as a clinical entity was strengthened by clinical descriptions, a survey [*Hall,* 1897] and the development of a lengthy list of descriptive terms covering the gamut of phobic phenomena.

When referring to phobic disorders we are not discussing the intense fearfulness which can be part of a melancholic or psychotic illness, nor are we discussing the realistic fear of a threatening external circumstance. If the fear of a loaded firearm pointing in one's direction lies at one end of a spectrum of fears, and the terror associated with the delusional belief that one is condemned for having committed the unpardonable sin at the other, the phobic disorders and panic under discussion here lie somewhere between those extremes and reflect a disproportionate response to a wholly imagined or exaggerated threat associated with a specific object, idea, or situation. The patient is aware of the irrationality of his reaction which remains inaccessible to logical argument, is involuntary, and is strengthened by the repeated avoidance of any contact with the provocative object or situation. It is a well-established finding that many phobic symptoms respond to the techniques of behavior modification better than they do to other forms of therapy [*Agras,* 1972] and that the use of hypnosis appears to enhance the effectiveness of behavioral methods.

Psychoanalytic theory, in essence, attributes phobias to a splitting off of the offending affect from an unacceptable idea, and its transference to an apparently harmless object, situation or notion [*Nemiah,* 1975]. The patient is then left with an awareness of a previously innocuous object, situation or idea now associated with a painful affect. As an example, the anxiety formerly belonging to a sexual thought that is no longer conscious could be transferred to an animal whose close presence would then be productive of what seemed to be senseless anxiety – a dog phobia for instance. This new object is then capable of stirring up the whole accumulation of feelings. By evading it the patient is usually able to escape the disabling anxiety. Anxiety related to separation, aggression and other primitive drives might also contribute to the formation of phobic behavior.

The principle underlying psychodynamic psychotherapy of phobic disorders is that psychological exploration enables the patient to discover the original conflict, and work at resolving it. This then liberates the symbolic situation or object from the anxiety that had been forced on it. It was acknowledged fairly early, however, that action was a necessary part of the successful therapy of phobias.

Learning theory supplies simple and intelligible explanations of several aspects of phobic symptoms. It has been repeatedly observed that a usually innocuous situation may become associated with anxiety if paired with a traumatic event. Furthermore, after witnessing a serious automobile accident or being thrown from a horse, a person might repeatedly avoid similar circumstances in the future. Those who assiduously avoid riding in an automobile or mounting a horse after such exposures will often, eventually, suffer a car phobia or horse-riding phobia that can persist for years. The current theories lead us to believe that the fear conditioned by the traumatic experience in these instances cannot undergo extinction because the behavior of avoiding riding in cars or horse-riding is being constantly reinforced and therefore maintained by the resulting reduction of anxiety. In patients with a more symbolic fear such as that of riding in an elevator, experience has repeatedly shown that those who succumb to the fear and either refuse to enter the elevator, or who leave it before their intended destination because of mounting fear and tension, experience an immediate abatement of anxiety as soon as they turn away from the elevator or begin to approach the staircase in preference. This avoidance response strengthens the conditioned avoidance (the elevator phobia).

The mechanisms by which the treatment methods of learning therapy work are not entirely clear, and differences of opinion exist. Although the mechanism in desensitization is thought by some to be counter-conditioning, that is, replacing an anxiety response with relaxation, others suggest that perhaps neither counter-conditioning nor a graduated approach are as important as the exposure to the feared situation itself. The therapeutic ingredient might well be habituation of the patient to the situation or object evoking the fear.

A Clinical Perspective

As indicated above, when hypnosis is used in conjunction with techniques aimed at replacing anxiety with relaxation, the therapeutic gains appear to be enhanced. The following case history is illustrative:

A man in his mid-20s who had been in traditional psychotherapy in the past, sought hypnosis because of his fear of dentistry. This fear had so crippled him that he had avoided seeing a dentist for over 10 years apart from one occasion when an infected impacted wisdom tooth drove him to seek help. He was remarkably responsive to hypnosis, scoring very high on the hypnotizability rating scales. On emerging from the experience of the induced trance, he volunteered the comment that it had felt not unlike what he remembered of his childhood experiences in the dentist's chair. He referred to feelings of dissociation in his head and limbs, and to his total preoccupation with particular parts of his body; all other stimuli were completely excluded. He was also able to make rapid use of strong hypnotic suggestions that he would be totally relaxed in the dentist's office and would experience only tingling and numb sensations in his jaw.

Other patients in describing phobic symptoms have also used phraseology not unlike that used by subjects who have had intense hypnotic experiences. They have talked of being able to observe themselves with some objectivity and of realizing the absurdity or irrationality of the situation. These reports have contributed to the idea that the events are possibly related. That, in fact, the essence of the phobic experience is not unlike that of the event of hypnosis, and that, perhaps, the phobic experience is in large measure a spontaneously occurring trance or dissociative experience similar to that which follows a hypnotic induction procedure. If this is so, it would require that phobic patients be, on average, more hypnotizable than others.

This was demonstrated by comparing the hypnotizability scores of a series of 24 phobic patients with those of an equal number of smokers who applied for treatment in hypnosis to relinquish the habit [*Frankel and Orne,* 1976]. The mean score of the phobics was 8.08 on a 12-point scale. The mean of the smokers was 6.08. The difference was significant beyond the 0.01 level (two-tailed). 30% of the smokers were non-responsive to hypnosis. This figure represents the percentage of nonresponders in any randomly chosen group of people. No phobic patients were nonresponsive. They were all at least moderately if not highly hypnotizable, and those with multiple phobias scored more highly than those with a single phobia.

A Theoretical View

These findings above should come as no great surprise to us. Clinicians at the turn of the century and earlier described a close association between high responsivity to hypnosis and the manifestation of hysterical symptoms [*Charcot,* 1886; *Janet,* 1907]. In fact, some considered hysteria to be equivalent to a spontaneous hypnotic event, one that took place in the absence of a formal induction procedure. More recent investigations [*Shor,* 1960; *Ås* et al., 1962] have proided the evidence that highly hypnotizable persons do indeed have personal experiences containing elements of the trance more frequently than poor responders.

These findings thus strongly support the notion that phobic patients show a tendency to the same kind of mental functioning that is involved in responding to a hypnotic induction. They must have the capability of manifesting the kind of cognitive functioning that characterizes the hypnotized individual. This implies the kind of mental process where images and fantasies can become sufficiently vivid and real as to be confused with the world outside, incongruities cease to be troublesome, logic can become temporarily superfluous, present experience takes precedence over the past and future, and a sense of time ceases to be important.

Recognizing, therefore, that the phobic patient's propensity for spontaneously occurring trance phenomena may provide the context for the symptoms to emerge, how can we adapt that information to the psycho-analytic or psychodynamic model? I believe it is possible to do so by viewing the spontaneous trance as a defense mechanism, in this case the maladaptive defense of dissociation. To elaborate, this means that the individual struggling with intolerable anxiety associated with an inadmissible idea or very disturbing situation containing intense rage, separation, or other affect, will resort to the defense of dissociation; this because of its nature, adds to rather than detracts from the anxiety. Panic might ensue and become firmly associated in the mind of the patient with the idea, situation, or object being encountered. In this way he learns to be fearful not only of the real situation or object, but even of the thought of it. By the constant evasion, the conditioned response of anxiety is reinforced.

An Integrative Approach to Treatment

Once one recognizes the phobic patient's propensity for spontaneously occurring trance phenomena, the experience of hypnosis might provide the means of helping the patient learn to understand more about the special mode of functioning that represents one of his assets as well as one of his liabilities [*Frankel,* 1976]. The state of hypnosis can provide the context in which to conduct an accelerated program of imaginal desensitization, or it may be used to produce an analogous symptom in the office that closely resembles the psychopathologic abnormalities most troublesome to the individual. If one can produce the symptoms and guide the patient to a degree of familiarity with and mastery over this very compelling but experimentally induced situation, he begins to learn something about the shift in functioning that is involved in causing and controlling his own psychopathological manifestations. At times the trance process can help the patient experience feelings previously seen as frightening and ego alien as familiar, under his control, and perhaps even as comfortable.

The treatment depends heavily on the use of self-hypnosis and the patient's readiness to practice on his own what he learns in the office. All such programs are introduced only after an adequate psychiatric evaluation of the clinical problem, with special attention focused on the psychodynamic understanding of its genesis and the degree of secondary gain. During the treatment, the patient has an opportunity to understand its origins both *psychodynamically* and *behaviorally,* and to master it. In essence, he learns to utilize the trance as a coping mechanism; this is accomplished within the framework of a psychodynamically sensitive treatment plan.

Furthermore, this application of hypnosis might be helpful within the context of current efforts aimed at investigating the use of short-term dynamic psychotherapy in chronically obsessive patients with multiple phobias [*Davanloo,* 1980] and in selected borderline patients [*Leibovich,* personal commun., 1979]. By the exclusion of cases that demonstrate the maladaptive defense described above, the application of traditional short-term dynamic psychotherapy can be focused with greater precision and the task of the therapist facilitated.

References

Agras, W.S.: in Agras, Behavior modification: principles and clinical applications (Little, Brown, Boston 1972).

Ås, A.; O'Hara, J.W; Munger, M.P.: The measurement of subjective experiences presumably related to hypnotic susceptibility. Scand. J. Psychol. *3:* 47–64 (1962).

Charcot, J.M.: Œuvres complètes (Progrès Médical, Paris 1886).

Davanloo, H.: Paper presented at the Workshop on Short-Term Dynamic Psychotherapy (Directors, *H. Davanloo; P.E. Sifneos*), Beth Israel Hospital, Harvard Medical School (June, 1980).

Diamond, M.J.: Modification of hypnotizability. A review. Psychol. Bull. *81:* 180–198 (1974).

Frankel, F.H.: Hypnosis: trance as a coping mechanism (Plenum Medical Book Company, New York 1976).

Frankel, F.H.; Orne, M.T.: Hypnotizability and phobic behavior. Archs gen. Psychiat. *33:* 1259–1261 (1976).

Hall, Y.S.: A study of fears. Am. J. Psychol. *8:* 147–249 (1897).

Hilgard, E.R.: Hypnotic susceptibility (Harcourt, Brace & World, New York 1965).

Hilgard, J.: Personality and hypnosis. A study of imaginative involvement (University of Chicago Press, Chicago 1970).

Janet, P.: The major symptoms of hysteria (Macmillan, New York 1907).

Leibovich, M. Personal commun. (1979).

Mesmer, F.A.: Mémoire sur la découverte du magnétisme animal (Geneva 1774).

Nemiah, J.C.: Phobic neurosis; in Freedman, Kaplan, Sadock, Comprehensive textbook of psychiatry/ii, vol. i, pp. 1231–1241 (Williams & Williams, Baltimore 1975).

Orne, M.T.: The nature of hypnosis. Artifact and essence. J. abnorm. soc. Psychol. *58:* 277–299 (1959).

Shor, R.E.: The frequency of naturally occurring 'hypnotic-like' experiences in the normal college population. Int. J. clin. exp. Hypn. *8:* 151–163 (1960).

Shor, R.E.: Three dimensions of hypnotic depth. Int. J. clin. exp. Hypn. *10:* 23–38 (1962).

Fred H. Frankel, MBChB, DPM, Department of Psychiatry, Beth Israel Hospital, Boston, Mass. (USA)

Psychother. Psychosom. *35:* 244–256 (1981)

Psychoanalysis and Brief Psychotherapy: Some New Considerations on the Psychotherapeutic Process

Edmond Gilliéron

Policlinique psychiatrique universitaire, Lausanne, Suisse

Key Words. Short-term dynamic psychotherapy · Psychoanalysis · Process

Abstract. This introductory paper describes the technique of brief analytic psychotherapy as has been developed in Lausanne. The author has tried to demonstrate that a single modification of the setting in comparison with psychoanalysis stresses the importance of the 'hic et nunc' in the therapeutic relationship. If this phenomenon becomes apparent to the therapist and is adequately interpreted, a natural associative process can develop where the analysis of transference and countertransference takes a primordial place. This process is comparable to psychoanalysis as far as certain transference movements are concerned, but the working mechanisms are different.

Introduction

Recently, I was introduced to a colleague as a 'Psychoanalyst specialising in brief psychotherapy'. He responded: 'Well, you are one of those therapists who are supposed to do in two months, what I need five years to complete.' I became a bit angry and I turned the discussion by saying: 'Well, you remind me of a man who denied the possibility of going from Boston to Montreal by plane in one hour, because he could walk in one month.' I am inclined to think that we often make similar mistakes: confusion between effects and means. You can arrive at the same destination; the point of arrival is the same, but the route is different, and what you see during the journey is different. I think that in the psychoanalytic field the major part of the criticisms of brief psychotherapy is influenced by two factors: (1) difficulty in distinguishing clearly between the psychotherapeutic and the psychoanalytic process, and (2) multiplicity of brief techniques, some of them having no clear frame of reference. My purpose is to propose a new way of studying the psychoanalytic psychotherapeutic process.

Confronted with the numerous forms of brief analytic psychotherapy that have developed since *Ferenczi's* field experiments [1918], most authors seek a better specificity of intervention, but in terms of patients' selection criteria: how to select a technique suitable for the patient. However, I am not sure that this way of questioning is right. Probably as *Luborsky* et al. [1975] say: 'Everyone has won and all must have prizes.' This means that there are different roads to the same destination. Therefore, we should look for a model that might explain why different methods have similar results. 'By a model we mean a frame of reference constructed in advance and involving a set of variables. The advantage of a model lies in the opportunity it offers to make comparisons necessary to all scientific generalisations' [*Gilliéron* et al., 1980]. Consequently, in order to overcome the difficulties emerging from the comparison between different kinds of brief analytic psychotherapy, psychoanalysis, and other doctor-patient relationships, I have proposed to leave aside the problem of selection criteria, as well as the one of results. A number of studies have already pointed out the importance of the nature of the patient-therapist relationship, for instance *Schneider* [1976] in the field of medical psychology, or *Malan* [1963, 1973] in therapeutic results.

My aim is twofold: to distinguish psychotherapy from a non-psychotherapeutic relationship, and to distinguish analytic psychotherapy from psychoanalysis. I have studied various situations: relationships between general practitioners and their patients, initially in the same way *Balint* did, and then by pointing out the influence of the family [*Gilliéron,* 1980]; relationships established by young medical students with a large variety of patients and seen in a large number of live interviews watched through a one-way mirror. In this way we could observe separately the *verbal* communications and the *non-verbal* ones: psychotherapies, psychoanalysis.

I have tried to understand how people behave in different situations as is shown in figure 1.

At one point I hit upon the very simple idea that, by doing this, I was defining psychotherapy as a particular situation; I was therefore more interested in the situation that defines psychotherapy, than in the psychotherapist's technique. Consequently, the psychotherapist's activity seemed to me less important than the situation, within the context of this activity. The first task is to define the influence of the frame of reference (or setting) on a relationship; the second is to determine how psychological change arises

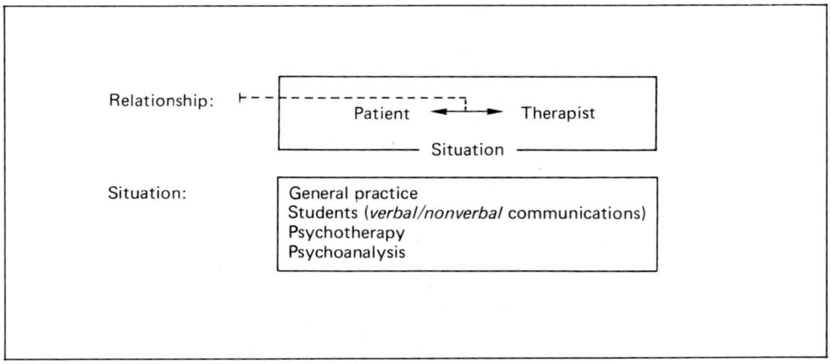

Fig. 1. Context (situation) and relationship.

within a relationship. From my point of view, psychoanalytic theory and the systemic model have been taken as frames of reference which may be seen as complementary [*Gilliéron,* 1979]. We can try to understand different parts of psychoanalytic work in the same way. We may then consider patient-therapist relationship as a whole in interaction where the patient has a significant influence on the therapist, as well as the therapist on the patient. In addition, both are influenced by the *context* of their action. Figure 2 partially summarizes these ideas: this diagram does not pretend to reflect all the subtleties of psychoanalytic treatment, but it is an attempt at a model which leads to an understanding of the important points at work in any psychotherapeutic process.

Figure 2 shows the following points: (1) The setting influences both patient and therapist. (2) There are two main channels of communication: verbal and nonverbal (visual perception). (3) The channel of visual perception is shorter than the one of verbalisation. (4) The relationship is a circular one. (5) The associations are the product of two main sources: influence of the therapist, inner problems. (6) Interpretations have two main sources: influence of the patient's associations, and a sum of personal factors (countertransference, technique, etc.).

I will not develop theoretical issues, but I will try to show a few aspects of our work, mainly: influence of the setting and its consequences on our technique.

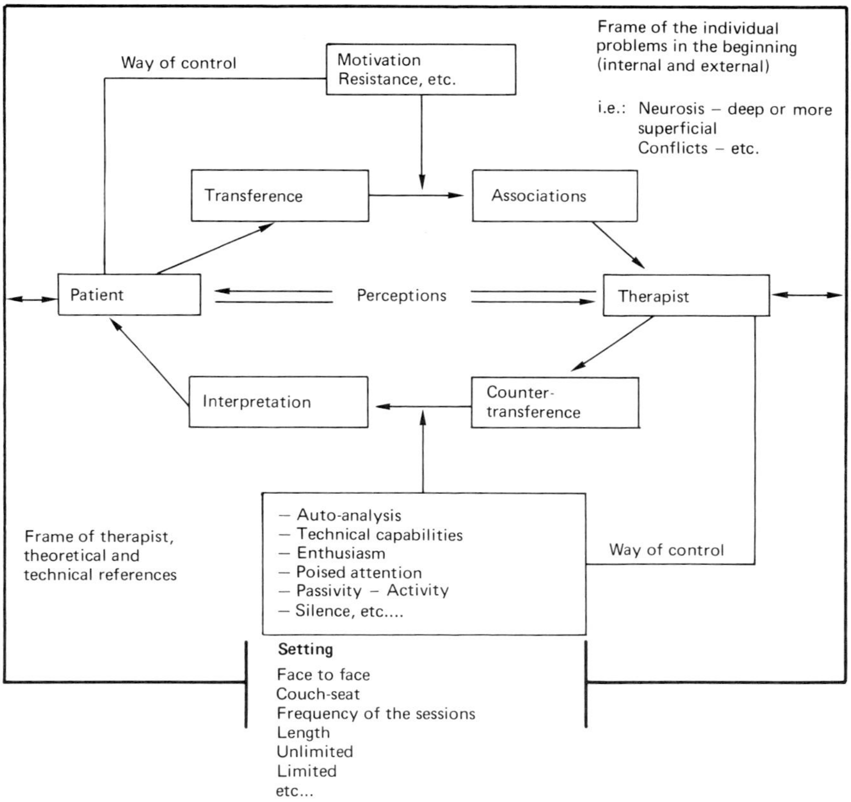

Fig. 2. Interaction patient-therapist.

About the Problems of Context: the Setting

Bateson [1980, p. 17] says about biology: ‘It is the context and it must surely be the receiving context that provides meaning for genetic instructions.’ My premise is an extrapolation of this point of view: I assume that the context provides meaning for the development of the therapy. In fact, I think that the terms of the context of the therapy should be considered as organising elements of the psychotherapeutic field, such as in any organised

Table I. Short-term psychotherapies

	Psycho-analysis	*Sifneos* [1972]	*Malan* [1963]	*Mann* [1973]	*Gilliéron and Premet* [in press]
Setting					
Relation	couch	facing	facing	facing	facing
Time-limit	none	limited, till major change	limited	limited strictly	limited strictly
Weekly sessions	regularly 3–5	regularly 1	regularly 1–2	regularly 1–2	regularly 1–2
Technique					
Therapist's attitude	neutral	'emotionally involved teacher'	senior lecturer'	'empathic helper'	neutral
Inter-ventions	nonselective, abstinence	selective attention-neglect	selective attention-neglect	selective attention	nonselective, abstinence
Emphasis	all asso-ciations	focus	focus	focus	all asso-ciations
Patient selection	flexible standards	rigid standards	more flexible standards	flexible standards	flexible standards

society, exchanges take place within culturally defined limits (national frontiers, family, school, etc.; school is the place where you learn, family where you grow, etc.).

The setting is the main part of the context in psychotherapy. I call setting the fixed data in the cure: frequency of sessions, time-limits, face-two-face, couch, etc. I call relationship anything taking place between the therapist and his patient, particulary the nature of the exchanges (free associations, interpretations, supportive interventions, etc.).

We might adopt the following axiom: the function of the setting is to establish a therapeutic field. This function is double. (a) To give meaning:

what happens in this office, during this period of time, etc., is of therapeutic nature. (b) To influence both therapist and patient in such a way that therapeutic work is possible. We might understand the influence of the setting on the mental functioning by comparing psychoanalysis and a few methods of brief psychotherapy in table I.

Table I shows the tendency to an increase in activity in brief psychotherapies, whereas in our technique, we do not modify our therapeutic attitude (behaviour) from that of psychoanalysis. We only take into account the modifications of the setting (*time-limit* and particulary *face to face*) and allow the patient to lead his treatment. But we are very attentive to the problem of interpretation as I will show.

We have to study the influence of different settings on different processes. That is, we might ask ourselves what we could bring out by changing the setting of the psychoanalytic process (couch, face to face) and by examining the patient-therapist relationship as a whole. In general we have to be aware of the influence of the setting on both the therapist's and the patient's mental functioning.

In another paper [*Gilliéron,* 1981], I have tried to show, as far as brief psychotherapies are concerned, the importance of two conditions of the setting: the limitation of time and the face to face technique. I have pointed out the fact that limitation of time is connected with the *economic point of view* in the psychoanalytic theory; the face to face with the rule of abstinence. Both conditions modify the psychoanalytic process in different but complementary ways: the time limit increases the emotional tension in the therapy, the face to face increases the involvement of both therapist and patient in such a way that it is much more difficult for both of them to ascertain the difference between transference and reality: the use of a face to face technique, since it brings the therapist into the patient's field of vision, creates a new therapeutic field where the person to person relationship seems to play a fundamental role.

Consequently, the latter situation leaves less room to the patient's imagination: as he sees his therapist, he tends to believe that he knows him. The fantasmatic field is thus reduced; this fact may explain a number of reactions against many psychotherapies: a defensive countertransferential reaction provoked by the fear of acting. If face to face leads to a confusion between unconscious fantasy and reality, the psychotherapist, in spite of his own didactic analysis, is also less prepared to differentiate his own feelings from the ones mobilised by the unconscious desires of the patient. These issues may be illustrated by the following example.

In a psychoanalytical setting (couch)

Patient:	'You are very depressed today.'
Therapist:	'Where does this feeling come from?'
Patient:	'I *saw* your face as I *came* in.'

In a psychotherapeutic setting (face to face)

Patient:	'You are very depressed today'.
Therapist:	'Where does this feeling come from?'
Patient:	'I *see* your face, *now:* I see that you really are very depressed today!'

This short example illustrates the importance of the setting: the fundamental difference between the couch transference-relationship and the face to face is that in the couch relationship the therapist and patient are speaking about memory: the affect may be present, but the representation based on perception clearly comes from the past; for example; what the patient saw when he entered, but what he does not see at present. In face to face, patient and therapist may think that they are talking about something that is happening now: the patient sees the therapist's face now and may believe that his perception is true. This example shows that one of the main difficulties in psychotherapy will be the constant confusion between fantasy and reality. This leads us to the second point of this paper: the patient-therapist relationship, their reciprocal influence, and the problem of the interpretation in a psychotherapeutic setting.

Therapeutic Relationship and Interpretation

In all types of psychotherapy, the setting must be clearly defined. Its function is to set the boundaries of the therapeutic field and to give both patient and therapist the possibility of therapeutic action. Corollarily, any therapist will find it difficult to get the slightest therapeutic change if the setting is not defined. I have often observed that such a setting is simply implicit, based on a tacit agreement between therapist and patient. I will try to demonstrate that the fundamentals of the interpretation are identical in psychotherapy and in psychoanalysis, but that the modifications of some terms of the setting impose a bigger effort by the therapist to understand the transference movements. I will illustrate some aspects of resistance in face to face relationship, how they affect the countertransference, and some solutions allowing a strict analytic approach.

The psychoanalytic method is linked to two basic concepts: the rules of abstinence and interpretation. I will show that it is much more difficult to abide by the rule of abstinence in psychotherapy.

In 1918, with *Ferenczi,* technical problems posed by the rule of abstinence came to the front of psychoanalytic debate and led to brief analytic techniques, based on a therapist's greater activity. According to our point of view, in the face to face relationship, the possibility given to the patient of seeing his therapist might be considered only as a way of modifying the nature of the therapeutic relationship. We have to understand and differentiate the following aspects. (1) The reciprocal influence on therapist-patient in the new setting, leading to a specific resistance: a power struggle between therapist and patient due to a misunderstanding of transference movements. (2) The specific way in which the patient's transference arises in face to face and the therapist's reactive countertransference. (3) The connection between behaviour and verbal language and the impact of the therapist's interpretations. These issues deal with the function of fantasmatic activity and symbolisation in the patient-therapist transactions.

Reciprocal Influence: the Power Struggle

The power struggle is strongly linked to the face-to-face situation. It may be illustrated by an example of an analytic psychotherapy of a female patient. This is a sequence of three sessions.

Clinical Example (The Psychotherapist Is a Training Analyst).

First session. We see the female patient talking a lot about her everyday life without showing any emotional involvement. The therapist tells her that she is resisting against the therapeutic process by controlling her affect, and says that if it goes on like this, the treatment probably will be useless.

Second session. Fruitful session during which the patient often burst into tears; she talked about childhood memories that she links with her present life. The therapist, after the session, is enthusiastic and says that prognosis is good.

Third session. The patient is depressed, and says that she wonders whether she should continue the treatment. The therapist gives the following interpretation: 'You wish to stop because you are afraid of loosing control of your emotions if you go on with the treatment.' The patient decides to continue.

In this interpretation we can see several metapsychological levels. An attempt to explain the feelings of the patient (she is anxious to loose control). A second explanation: the treatment pushes the patient to give up this control. Thirdly, an implicit order: 'Stay, don't leave.'

Here we observe the struggle between patient and therapist. In the first session the therapist indirectly threatens to abandon her if she keeps on with her behaviour. The second session: the patient obeys her therapist by showing affect and the therapist is glad. The third session: the patient is depressed and asks implicitly: 'I have done what you asked and what will you do for me now.' The therapist's interpretations may be considered as an expression of his desire to keep the patient in a nonverbal way. There is a not mentioned transference-countertransference relationship. The resistance of both patient and therapist concerning their own affective involvement results from a confusion between fantasy and reality. The therapist is inclined to believe that he really wants to keep the patient as a person. In such a situation some questions arise.

If the therapist had only said: 'Stay!' would it have been as powerful? I don't think so. This simple fact shows the impact of the nonverbal aspect in the therapy since there is no possibility of arguing. The communication is direct, unequivocal, fairly unconscious and thus very strong. Language has an ambiguous and interposing function in a relationship; it allows discussion and implicitly alternatives.

In our example the only solution of the problem is insight into the situation. In fact we have to investigate where do the fantasies originate in interactions. In this transference-countertransference relationship, both therapist and patient behave as if there was a conflict-situation. There is no room for discussion about the roots of their behaviour in the transference relationship, nor about the connections with the patient's images, etc. They are talking about something they are not aware about, and they behave in a struggling way. Paradoxically, the therapist's behaviour is an acting-out.

If, in the third session, he had just said something like this: 'In the last session, you showed a lot of your feelings, perhaps a bit in order to please me, now you seem afraid to expect something more from me', they could thus have the possibility of discovering the underlying fantasies. I shall refer to this subject later by discussing the connections between behaviour and language.

Transference and Countertransference (Resistance by Transference)

A close relationship implies behavioural rules such as cultural habits that keep up the cohesion of the group. In psychotherapy you can take advantage in considering that rules (such as the rule of abstinence) have a unique therapeutic function. The resistance by transference might be considered as a transgression of therapeutic rules. Let us consider the following example.

In a psychotherapeutic sequence, the therapist clearly perceives in a female patient's associations an oedipal conflict. He has the opportunity to give a clear but partial interpretation which is well accepted by the patient, who starts to speak about her past frustrations. The therapist feels very satisfied. Suddenly, the patient stops and says: 'Everything we are talking about is useless. I thought you were able to help me, but you are only interested in my past, not in my present life. What I need is direct interest and active help.' The therapist gets very embarrassed and answers that the patient's remarks are very important; he shortens the session and proposes to talk about it in the next one.

The therapist would have been less embarrassed if he had understood that the patient was attacking his therapeutic function and the rule of abstinence, whose purpose is to give rise to unconscious fantasies and memories. Whereas unconsciously he shared the patient's beliefs and became anxious. This reaction is frequently seen in psychotherapy. Either example shows the difficulty of interpreting fantasies in a face to face relationship. A way of understanding activity-passivity problems and the place of language in a relationship will be illustrated in the next vignette.

Verbal and Nonverbal Communication (Introducing Meaning into a Relationship)

This example comes from a nonpsychotherapeutic doctor-patient relationship, which will illustrate the problems posed by behavioural resistance which is more characteristic of the face to face situation. I will try to show a way of respecting the rule of abstinence that facilitates interpretation. A female patient, 60 years old, is sent to a psychiatrist by her surgeon, because she is depressed after a cancer operation. The psychiatrist is confronted with a strong and manipulative patient who asks many questions, not listening to what he is telling her. He realises that she controls the relationship and that talking about her fears and her problems is impossible. This patient has been a strong woman who, since her childhood, took care of her paralysed mother and (afterwards) a husband that was always ill. Her first illness was cancer, and after a short moment of depression, she denied any difficulty. This patient, who had to overcome many problems in her life, had lived with a certain sense of omnipotence. She never could expect support from anybody; she always had to support others. With the doctors she repeated this behaviour in a defensive way, denying depression and illness. On this problem, discussion between patient and therapist was possible via activity or abstinent-passive orientation. An active doctor could have shown his patient her denial but in doing so a struggle against resistance would have started. An abstinent-passive doctor could have accepted the patient's behaviour and would say something like this: 'Many doctors have tried to help you without success. I see that we are also unable to help you in the proper way. You have always been a strong woman, able to take care of yourself and of others. I don't know what to do.' In doing this, the doctor would have openly accepted the patient's projective identification. But he would have left her the possibility of answering: 'You are like the others, nobody has ever helped me in my life and now you will not help me either.' The possibility to talk about psychological problems would have been introduced in the relationship, without any form of activity but with something based on an interpretation.

Probably, in the long run, the two attitudes would have the same results, but the second one is more powerful. Such an intervention is closely linked to *Freud's* description of the first stages of the mother-child relationship. In his book 'Interpretation of Dreams', he says that the infant, in a situation of frustration, replaces the absent breast by a hallucination. Surprisingly, psychoanalysts did not pay enough attention to the implications of that concept. In the Freudian idea, the fantasmatic process can replace for a moment the libidinal satisfaction. The construction of the fantasmatic world is based on two experiences: satisfaction and frustration. This Freudian reconstruction implies a connection between a double behaviour: that of the mother and that of the child, as well as the mental life. I am not sure that what *Freud* described was really what happens in the infant's mind, but I am certain what he discovered there is an important issue in the mental functioning. He discovered that a human being can think and imagine rather than either acting or fulfilling his libidinal needs in a broad sense.

Thus, in the latter way of dealing with the patient, we may say that the therapist brings in frustration and consequently the imagery dimension. He would disappear as a person if he accepted the patient's projection; in so doing, he would frustrate any patient's libidinal needs. So she would not need to use her resistance movements, she would only have recourse to her inner imagos: 'You are like the others (in my past), you don't help me!' 'The others' about whom she speaks are people in the past, memories. And the work of interpretation becomes possible: hate towards bad objects, etc.

Summary

Summarizing, I have tried to show: the need for a clear distinction between the specific effects bound to the context or setting, and those bound to the technique of intervention (interpretations, for example) in the therapeutic relationship; the necessity to consider the patient-therapist relationship itself as a dynamic, circular one, in which each participant influences the other; and the necessity to determine the respective position of fantasies and behaviour in any therapeutic relationship.

In three examples we have seen some movements that are more characteristic of psychotherapy: (1) the power struggle that might be considered as a resistance against transference; (2) a transference reaction that might be considered as a resistance against memories; (3) the psychotherapist's tendency towards activity that might be considered as a result of his difficulty in reaching awareness of the fantasies underlying the patient's behaviour. I assume that in these cases, the analyst's difficulties are strongly related to the face to face situation and the consecutive risk of confusion between transference and reality. Neither the patient nor the therapist are fully aware of the projective mechanisms. This situation may lead to subtle acting out on the part of the analyst which are hidden behind interpretations.

References

Bateson, G.: Mind and nature. A necessary unity (Bantam Books, New York 1980).

Gilliéron, E.: Psychanalyse et système sont-ils inconciliables? Le processus psychothérapique. Eléments d'un modèle; dans Co-thérapie et co-thérapeutes. Association des méthodes en psychothérapie. Annales de psychothérapie, pp. 61–73 (ESF, Paris 1979).

Gilliéron, E.: Influence of the setting on a psychotherapeutic relationship in analytically oriented brief psychotherapy. Psychother. Psychosom. *35:* 44–54 (1981).

Gilliéron, E.: Le médecin praticien et la famille. Folia psychopract. (1980).

Gilliéron, E.; Leresche, G.; Bovet, J.: Trial models of the psychotherapeutic process; in de Moor, Wijngaarden, Psychotherapy: research and training, pp. 87–90 (Elsevier/North-Holland Biomedical Press, Amsterdam 1980).

Gilliéron, E.; Premet, I.: Introduction aux psychothérapies brèves d'inspiration psychanalytique. Archs Suisses Psychiat. Neurol. Neurochir. (in press).

Luborsky, L.; Singer, B.; Luborsky, L.: Comparative studies of psychotherapies. Is it true that 'Everyone has won and all must have prizes?'. Archs gen. Psychiat. *32:* 995–1008 (1975).

Malan, D.: A study of brief psychotherapy (Tavistock Publications, London 1963).
Malan, D.: Therapeutic factors in analytically oriented brief psychotherapy; in Gosling, Support, innovation and autonomy (Tavistock Publications, London 1973).
Malan, D.: The frontier of brief psychotherapy (Plenum Medical Book Company, New York 1976).
Mann, J.: Time-limited psychotherapy (A Commonwealth Fund Book, Harvard University Press, Cambridge 1973).
Schneider, P.-B.: Propédeutique d'une psychothérapie (Payot, Paris 1976).
Sifneos, P.: Short-term psychotherapy and emotional crisis (Harvard University Press, Cambridge 1972).

Edmond Gilliéron, Médecin-chef, Policlinique psychiatrique universitaire, 26, rue St-Martin, CH–1005 Lausanne (Switzerland)

Psychother. Psychosom. *35:* 257–264 (1981)

Short-Term Psychotherapy for the Borderline Personality Disorder

Miguel A. Leibovich
Harvard Medical School, and Beth Israel Hospital, Boston, Mass., USA

Key Words. Short-term dynamic integrative psychotherapy · Borderline

Abstract. This paper presents concepts of short-term therapy as utilized with borderline personality disorder. Criteria for patient selection as well as contraindications for its use are presented. Many clinical symptoms are rubricated under borderline disorders. One major consideration in diagnosis is based on the discernment of when developmental arrests have occurred. The author's opinion is that short-term integrative psychotherapeutic procedures can be beneficial for patients struggling with any of the developmental subphases. The concepts expressed in this paper are mostly applicable to more developed individuals, who have progressed in differentiating themselves from others, but who still present primitive characteristics and relationships.

Introduction

The number of patients presenting a clinical picture with borderline pathology has increased markedly during the last 20 years. This is usually reported by clinicians working in out-patient as well as in-patient settings, emergency services and practitioners in private practice doing psychotherapy or psychoanalysis. The question of whether this is due to an increase in actual numbers of these patients, to clinicians' greater propensity to use this diagnostic category or the development of more precise diagnostic methods is not yet answered. The reality is that it is quite common to encounter a large patient population that shows fragile ego structures with severe and ominous symptomatology that require psychotherapeutic methods of a nature quite different from those used with the better-integrated individuals or neurotics. Some of these psychotherapeutic methods are: long-term psychoanalytically or behaviorally oriented psychotherapy; emergency approaches; crisis interventions; brief intermittent supportive therapeutic contacts with or without the utilization of psychotropic medication; group psychotherapy; and short-term psychotherapy. In discussions of short-term psychotherapy it has, in general, been assumed that ego-disorganized patients like borderline personalities, cannot profit from brief, understanding prompting, ego building, dynamically oriented treatment and that only quick supportive contacts on a crisis or long-term educative therapy are useful. In this paper I will suggest that for some purposes the utilization of short-term psychotherapy may be the treatment of choice for individuals exhibiting manifest borderline symptomatology or personality disturbances. More concretely, my discussion will be about the overall principles underlying the conceptualization of *short-term integrative psychotherapy* (STIP), the type of borderline patients for whom this method is suitable, and the clinical conditions in which it is contraindicated.

Short-Term Integrative Psychotherapy: General Principles

The basic theoretical concepts of short-term integrative psychotherapy are rooted in the principles of psychoanalytic developmental psychology, sometimes called ego psychology, and in object-relations theory.

The patients selected are struggling with emotional troubles, but are not necessarily in the midst of a decompensation. However, at times during treatment, a crisis situation may emerge. Occasionally, individuals appear in a state of emotional dyscontrol but may proceed with short-term therapy if they are able to overcome the critical period and commit themselves to more prolonged and exploratory psychotherapeutic work.

The goal of short-term integrative psychotherapy for borderlines is primarily to alleviate the distressing symptoms and to alter some of the maladaptive personality patterns. This is accomplished by assisting patients: (a) to become aware of their unrecognized dynamic distortions; (b) to correct their ego deficiencies and poor coping abilities, and (c) to discover and utilize their stable and constant ego functions. Throughout the therapy one of the emphases is on the strengthening of the ego functions which are laboring inadequately. Short-term integrative psychotherapy tends to be less centered on the historical past. Greater consideration is given to: (a) the current emotional troubles of the patient (the here and now); (b) the ongoing psychotherapeutic relationship and its fluctuations, and (c) the transference manifestations, especially negative, only if they happen to develop during this short period of treatment.

The empathic therapeutic framework and technique is based on our present knowledge of the importance of altered pre-oedipal relationships and ego deficiencies in the pathology of the borderline person. Special attention is paid to the problems stemming from an unresolved *separation-individuation phase* of psychological development. The working through of the complicated stages of that developmental period is the essential focus of short-term integrative psychotherapy. The work centers around the anxieties and insecurities surrounding the patient's fragile sense of *intrapsychic separateness* and *individuality*. The ego of the patient has become impaired. Attempts to heal the fragmented ego become the very fabric of this approach and its procedures must be designed specifically for that purpose. In my opinion, if a borderline patient enters psychotherapy for the first time, a short-term method should be attempted initially. Short-term therapy can be offered to borderline patients who have never had any psychiatric contacts, or patients who have had previous psychiatric encounters of various kinds: (a) exclusively psychotropic medications, electroconvulsive therapy or purely maintenance supportive interventions such as reassurance, approval, directiveness, suggestion, encouragement and praise without an attempt at developing a dynamic understanding of the psychological problems, or (b) psychotherapy which did not produce much symptom relief or personality changes, and (c) psychotherapeutic experiences that not only produced a stalemate but also caused unwelcome regressive phenomena.

A clinical vignette may illustrate this point. A 45-year-old divorced male was referred for a consultation to assess the possibility of short-term psychotherapy for his psychological difficulties. The diagnosis was borderline personality disturbance. Patient had functioned rather marginally in the area of interpersonal relationships despite significant scholastic achievements. At the time of the death of his divorced wife (7 years prior to the consultation) he had become more disorganized and was admitted to a psychiatric institution where he remained for 14 months. During this and other hospitalizations as well as outpatient psychiatric intervention, the patient was treated either with antidepressants, neuroleptics, or electroconvulsive therapy. Even during the current evaluation, he was receiving a weekly maintenance application of electroconvulsive therapy. Psychotherapy had been attempted but the techniques utilized did not render any favorable effects. This patient fulfilled the criteria for short-term integrative psychotherapy and was treated for 9 months, with a beneficial outcome.

Selection Criteria and Therapeutic Agreement

The selection of a person for short-term integrative psychotherapy is based on a tentative diagnostic appraisal of the patient's ego development in the present and in his life history. Of special significance are those areas as *love* (relationships) and *work* and how successfully developmental milestones like the phase of separation-individuation and its subphases (differentiation, practicing, rapprochement, and separation-individuation, per se) have been resolved. Then, from the rough data from this evaluation a tentative decision is reached about whether the patient falls into one of the three broad categories: neurotic, borderline or psychotic structure. More specifically, there are several essential factors in the selection of borderline patients for short-term integrative psychotherapy.

(1) *Evidence of sufficient reality testing* that would enable patients to commit their time, energy and money for approximately 6–9 months, for once or twice a week sessions, and engage themselves in a therapeutic agreement. The patient needs to understand that the therapeutic process will be a collaborative effort with the therapist.

(2) *Motivation:* patients have to manifest the wish for psychological help in order to change their maladaptive traits. They must show willingness to embark upon the exploratory process in order to correct what is not functioning well. Any expectations that results will be obtained without their active participation and have to be clarified and dispelled.

(3) Patients must exhibit some degree of *intrapsychic and emotional* separateness to the extent that they realistically will be able to accept the *distinctiveness* of the therapist that *there is another individual in the room* with them. The borderline patient's tendency to *psychically enmesh or fuse* should not be too strong, that is, his inclination to fall into interactional styles which would indicate a poorly resolved self-object differentiation should be moderate.

(4) Patient's ability to interact and to relate effectively with the therapist needs to be relatively preserved. There must be evidence of some *positive emotional connection* with the evaluator, of *rapport* which will favor the formation of a favorable therapeutic relationship and alliance.

(5) In assessing the borderline's past relationships there must be evidence of some warm, positive interactions; friendships even if superficial; a desire to connect with other people and the existence of relationships even if these were short lived, complicated and unsatisfactory. That is, the ego capacity for *having attempted* relationships must be present.

(6) It is also important to make a rapid assessment of what appears to be the borderline patient's *basic mood* in their past as well as present life. *Mahler* [1971] in studying the *separation-individuation period* of early childhood development described a characteristic affective responsiveness, a *basic mood* that presumably predisposes to certain emotional reactions in later life (depressive or anxiety spells, angry outbursts and boredom or on the other side of the affective continuum, elation, hypomanic excitement and a sense of omnipotence). A positive feature for the selection of patients for short-term integrative psychotherapy is a *basic mood* of contentment, a kind of overexcitement and a mild sense of overconfidence. This basic mood may reflect the borderline's somewhat positive emotional experience during the *practicing subphase* of development which left intact the stable ego processes which must be functional for this therapy to be effective.

(7) Patient's complicated ego function of *verbalization* must have developed sufficiently for him to be capable of enunciating (even if not entirely coherently) his current disturbances and emotional pains. If too chronic and pronounced fright and inhibitions produced thought and verbal blocking, short-term integrative psychotherapy would not be possible.

(8) The presence of stable and intact ego functions which assisted the borderline patient in achieving certain successes during his life is necessary. In adult borderline structures it is of significance to remember that almost never is the clinical situation one in which the patient is stagnant *at just one point of development*. So during the psychodiagnostic process for short-term therapy, the assessment includes: (a) the number and type of stable ego functions in operation; (b) the degree of ego modification; (c) the highest level of development reached, and (d) where the ego regression lies at the time of the evaluation. For this kind of therapy the borderline patient must still be struggling with *separation-individuation issues of development*. Conflict-free ego capabilities like perception, discipline, perseverance, desires for advancement, tenacity, etc. manifested through achievements in occupational, social, political, academic or familial spheres must be evident. Short-term integrative psychotherapy can be quite useful with individuals functioning well *only* in certain sectors (occupational or academic for example) while serious diffuculties exist in areas like interpersonal relationships, self-esteem or other ego developmental deviations. Average intelligence and the capacity for introspection are also, naturally, desirable characteristics. Examination of many patients labelled with the nosological category of borderline personality disorder shows that in some, certain ego functions will be *more* impaired while others remain constantly quite strong, intact and

stable. The precise discernment of these different patterns is fundamental for a favorable outcome of short-term integrative psychotherapy. The determination of the functions disrupted or fragmented currently and in the past guides the course and sets the goals of treatment. A common mistake is often made: the emphasis on the pathological aspects and the neglect of the strengths and healthy resources of the individual.

(9) Patients should have the capacity to recognize the *existence of a focal troublesome issue.* The therapist should be able during the first two interviews to identify a *central problematic* pattern or characteristic around which many of the patient's difficulties revolve. There should be congruence between patient and therapist about the validity as well as the relevance, in terms of the patient's life situation and priorities, of the focal issue selected for therapeutic work. This is the recognition and acceptance of the *core problem.* The *focus* with these patients could be: low tolerance for frustration and consequent explosive destructive behavior, weakened ability to delay immediate gratifications, tendency to develop rapid and entangled interactions and relationships, poor ability for psychic differentiation between self and others, diminished capacity to bear anxiety, depression or other unpleasant affects, tendency to externalization and projection of the *bad self-images,* high degree of *personalization* in human contacts, exaggerated manipulative traits in interactions, overdependency which stunts the utilization of the patient's own capabilities and resources, etc.

Other areas toward which *to focus* the therapy could be: the degree of troubles in the existing operative relationships with the environment, the reversing of the process of regressive infantile expectation for constant and total gratifications which often bring major disappointments with inappropriate anger and maladaptive behavior, the turning of the emotion of anger and its derivatives from an inward direction against the self or the working through of the polarized concept of the self between a *great-unique-magnificent one* and a *bad-awful-monstrous self.* Sometimes the therapeutic work can also find as a focus some of the borderline primitive defenses like: projective identification, omnipotence, avoidance through action, aggrandizement and devaluation, splitting, etc.

(10) Patients should have somewhat realistic expectations about the results of short-term psychotherapy. They must understand that changes may occur only in the areas agreed upon. If they insist upon unrealistic results, like major personality changes, from a psychotherapeutic involvement of forty to fifty weeks, they should be included in other therapeutic modalities.

Borderline patients with the following characteristics *should not be accepted* for short-term integrative psychotherapy. (a) Individuals in a severe state of dyscontrol, with marked impulsivity and destructive tendencies toward themselves or others. (b) Patients whose defenses like externalizations, denial, grandiosity, projection are *so fixed* that it is difficult to establish a realistic interaction with the therapist. (c) The constricted, *schizoid* type of borderline individual who is too withdrawn and verbalizes poorly with speech characterized by vagueness, prolonged silences, blocking or distractedness. (d) The absence of any current relationships or if these are only the original familial ones. (e) A severe but temporary break with reality manifested by hallucinations, delusions, etc. (f) The inability to accept the appropriate boundaries of the therapeutic setting, that is, patients whose reality sense is quite impaired and who may still be arrested at the *symbiotic phase* of development not permitting them to form a favorable therapeutic relationship, with the qualities of *mutuality*.

Sometimes, during the psychodiagnostic procedure, patients already show intense primitive reactions. One encounter illustrates this point: when a patient came for a second evaluation visit, she went to my private study and began looking through my books. She did not go to the waiting area which was clearly designated. When I went to greet her I gently asked that the next time she wait for me in the waiting room. She reacted with unusual hostility to my remarks, began to scream, insulted me and said that she had to see the books to learn about my psychological orientation. She could not comprehend how I dared to tell her that she could not browse through my bookcase. After a brief discussion she could not accept my request. This intense reaction to not obtaining the gratification she wanted proceeded for the next few sessions until she finally settled down. Naturally, this patient was not accepted for short-term integrative psychotherapy.

Summary

This paper presents the overall concepts of short-term therapy as it is utilized with a certain group of people diagnosed as having a borderline personality disorder. There are many clinical symptoms that fall under the rubric of borderline disorders. It is an oversimplification to think of borderlines as exhibiting only one kind of clinical picture. One major consideration in the diagnosis of these patients is based on the discernment of when the developmental arrests have occurred. There are patients who have not progressed from the symbiotic phase of development, show a severe picture of borderline pathology but still are not psychotic. There are other borderline individuals who are still fixated at levels corresponding to the different subphases of the *separation-individuation phase* be it the *differentiation, practicing, rapprochement* or *separation-individuation proper* subphases. It is my opinion that short-term psychotherapeutic procedures can be beneficial for boderline patients still struggling with any of these developmental subphases. I wish to emphasize, however, that the concepts expressed in this paper are mostly applicable to the more developed borderline individuals. These are the patients who have progressed through the vicissitudes of psychically differentiating themselves from others, who have attained a certain mastery and competence (via their autonomous ego functions which have not been affected by major setbacks during the *practicing* subphase) but who, due to unresolved struggles in their reapprochement and separation-individuation periods, still present rather primitive characteristics and primitive human relationships. Short-term integrative psychotherapy can be useful for these individuals. The criteria for patient selection as well as contraindications for its use are presented in this paper.

References

Bellak, L.; Small, L.: Emergency psychotherapy and brief psychotherapy; 2nd ed. (Grune & Stratton, New York 1977).

Leibovich, M.; McGuire, M.T.: The use of intact ego functions in short-term psychotherapy. Proc. VIIth Int. Congr. Psychotherapy, Psychother. Psychosom., *15:* 1–46 (1967).

Leibovich, M.: Short-term adaptive psychotherapy. Proc. VIIth Int. Congr. Psychotherapy. Psychother. Psychosom. *15:* 1–38 (1967).

Leibovich, M.: An aspect of the psychotherapy of borderline personalities; in What is psychotherapy? Proc. IXth Int. Congr. Psychotherapy. Psychother. Psychosom. *25:* 53–57 (1975).

Leibovich, M.: Short-term psychotherapy for hysterical personalities. Stages of the therapeutic processes. Psychother. Psychosom. *24:* 67–78 (1974).

Leibovich, M.: Short-term psychotherapy for borderline patients. Course, Am. Psychiat. Ass. Meet., Chicago 1979.

Mahler, M.S.: A study of the separation-individuation process and its possible application to borderline phenomena in the psychoanalytic situation. Psychoanalyt. Study Child *26:* 403–425 (1971).

Miguel A. Leibovich, MD, Assistant Clinical Professor of Psychiatry, Harvard Medical School, Boston, Mass. (USA)

Psychother. Psychosom. *35:* 265–270 (1981)

Short-Term Dynamic Psychotherapy: Progress, Problems, Perspectives

Roland Pierloot

University of Leuven, Belgium

Key Words. Short-term dynamic psychotherapy · Hague Workshop

Abstract. The II Hague Workshop offered an opportunity to representants of the short-term dynamic psychotherapy to demonstrate and confront their techniques and theoretical assumptions. The principal results of this exchange of ideas, with regard to identity and differentiation of the therapy, evaluation of patients suitable for this therapy, therapeutic technique, assessment of outcome, suitability and training of the therapists, are summed up.

Introduction

The wealth of clinical material and theoretical assumptions concerning short-term dynamic psychotherapy, exposed in the II Hague Workshop can be summed up under these three headings: progress, problems and perspectives. These characteristics apply to different aspects of this psychotherapy form: (1) identity and differentiation of the therapy; (2) evaluation of patients suitable for this therapy; (3) therapeutic technique; (4) assessment of outcome, and (5) suitability and training of the therapist.

The essential contributions on each of these issues, emerging from the different papers and interventions during the workshop, are reflected in the following considerations.

Identity and Differentiation of Short-Term Dynamic Psychotherapy

In former publications the pioneers of short-term dynamic psychotherapy have described different forms of this technique, such as the short-term anxiety-provoking therapy for neurotic patients with unresolved oedipal problems [*Sifneos,* 1979], the brief psychotherapy for patients with more profound problems such as the resolution of morbid grief reactions [*Malan,* 1963, 1976b], the technique for more disturbed individuals such as those suffering from chronic obsessive illnesses and multiple phobias [*Davanloo,* 1978]. By introducing the short-term *integrative* therapy for borderline patients [*Leibovich,* 1980] and referring to some connections between hypnosis and short-term psychotherapy [*Frankel,* 1980], the scope of this therapy form has been broadened considerably.

This development is welcome and interesting, because one of the common objections against short-term dynamic psychotherapy has been that it can be used only for a very limited number of patients, mostly the less disturbed. Such a broader view on short-term dynamic psychotherapy also confronts us with the necessity to define on one hand the essential features of this therapy in general, and on the other hand some basis for the differentiation of several variants.

It is clear that *Frankel* [1980] does not call his technique of hypnosis a form of short-term *dynamic* psychotherapy. Still, in his theoretical representation of phobic behavior he is using psychoanalytic concepts such as the unconscious, intrapsychic conflict, anxiety, defenses and ego-integrative functions. By this way the experiences in his technique can be helpful to clarify the therapeutic process in forms of dynamic psychotherapy. This psychoanalytic model also underlies the different types of short-term dynamic psychotherapy, but it is combined with a number of practical criteria: the active and intensive use of the transference, the focal formulations and interpretations, the limited and circumscribed goals, the limitation of duration, the face to face setting.

If these are the specific characteristics of short-term dynamic psychotherapy, how can different forms be differentiated? Where should we look for the differences between the anxiety-provoking therapy of *Sifneos* [1979], the brief focal therapy of *Malan* [1976b], the special techniques described by *Davanloo* [1978] and *Gilliéron* [1980], and the integrative therapy of *Leibovich* [1980]? When we analyse their clinical material the most striking differences seem to emerge in the accenting of elements such as the breaking through of the resistances, the way of insisting on feelings and fantasy contents, the stressing of conflict-solving interpretations, the use of the setting and nonverbal elements, the part of the ego-strengthening function of the therapeutic alliance, the preparation for the end of the therapy, the importance of cognitive restructuring versus corrective emotional experience in the therapeutic process. The managing of these elements also has its repercussion on the choice of patients, considered as suitable for this therapy.

It will be an important task in the further development of short-term dynamic psychotherapy to clarify and delimitate in a more elaborate way the resemblances and differences between the variants of this therapeutic technique.

Evaluation of Patients Suitable for Short-Term Dynamic Psychotherapy

Criteria such as a chief complaint, possibilities of meaningful relationship, introspective capacities and psychological sophistication, flexibility of interaction, the definition of a focal conflict, willingness, motivation and realistic expectations, formulated by *Sifneos* [1979] and *Malan* [1976b] and extensively elaborated by *Davanloo* [1978] remain important guidelines. This applies also to the definition of some contraindications found in important acting-out behavior, impending psychosis, and real suicide planning.

Is an evaluation on such a basis too narrow, as has been suggested?

Leibovich [1980] provided a somewhat modified version, adapted to borderlines. *Davanloo* [1978] could demonstrate how important changes in the attitudes of the patient take place after the breaking through of strong resistances, especially against anger and aggression. Does not such an approach makes it possible to detect in the patient capacities and qualities seemingly absent before? This means that selection is dependent on the way of conducting the evaluation interview.

More and more the conviction grows that perhaps the most important criterion for selection can be found in the response of the patient to trial interpretations, particularly transference interpretations, in the evaluation interview. The use of this interview as a trial therapy has been suggested. The question arises if this could be harmful in some cases, making a preselection necessary.

Technique of Short-Term Dynamic Psychotherapy

The basic assumption that the therapeutic process is based on a combination of therapeutic alliance and transference experiences, leaves no doubt. The working alliance manifests itself in the agreement on a psychodynamic hypothesis, the time limits, the problem solving changes and the strengthening of ego-functions. The transference and the past-present links are the subjects of an intense interpreting working-through.

With regard to the handling of the resistances, different approaches have been demonstrated. *Sifneos* in his technique [1979] is more inclined to a gently undermining, a going behind the resistances, while *Davanloo* [1978] insists on challenging the resistances. *Gilliéron* [1980] presents a more classic psychoanalytic form of interpreting the resistances. There exists a general agreement that in this area a flexible attitude of the therapist, adapted to the type of patient and the phase of the treatment, is necessary. Focusing is essential in this technique, but the choice of a focal conflict can be a point of discussion. Although oedipal problems seem to fit the best in this technique, pre-oedipal conflicts should not be excluded. Abandonment-anxiety needs a thorough preparation of the end of the therapy [*Malan,* 1963]. In borderline patients, the separation-individuation conflict offers the best opportunities [*Leibovich,* 1980].

The pronounced insisting on an exhaustive representing of feelings and fantasies demands an active engagement of the therapist. Such an attitude results in the production of a rich material by the patient but the question arises in how far this attitude offers the danger of promoting countertransference reactions. These can be of an aggressive or erotic nature. Fear of such countertransference reactions can perhaps explain the reluctance of some therapists against this therapeutic techniques.

Other aspects of the technique, such as the face to face and time-limited setting, and the importance of nonverbal manifestations, stressed by *Gilliéron* [1980], can open new perspectives in the further elaboration of the technique.

Assessment of Outcome

With a therapy directed to limited, circumscribed goals, evaluation of the outcome should be easier than with classic psychoanalysis, aiming at a general growth and maturation of personality. There seems to exist an agreement that the expectated outcome should be formulated in terms of concrete, and for each individual specific, attitudes, feelings and behavior patterns, based on a psychodynamic formulation of the focal problem(s). Disturbing manifestations must not only disappear but they should be replaced by more constructive solutions.

In the procedure of assessment different variants can be used. Who should evaluate? The patient, the therapist, a neutral evaluator or a combination of these possibilities? When should the evaluation take place; at the end of the therapy or after a certain interval? The role of the environment and its inevitable interaction with the changes in the patient should not be neglected. This means that differences can occur between the results at the end of the therapy and at a later date.

Although some problems cannot be denied, the outcome studies by *Sifneos* [1979], *Malan* [1976a] and *Davanloo* (1978) offer interesting prospects. In the study of *Meyer* [1980] the attention has been drawn to the relation between focus formulation and outcome. An often repeated question concerns the comparison of the results of short-term and long-term psychodynamic psychotherapy. A reliable study would offer important difficulties: not only the patients but also the therapists must be similar.

Suitability and Training of the Therapist

Not enough time could be devoted to the issue of the suitability and training of the therapist. *Heiberg* [1980] exposed the importance of a research-oriented organisation, the intervision in groups of therapists and the modelling from a guest professor. Other interesting subjects for discussion could be the possible selection of candidates, the opportunity of a general psychoanalytic training, the modalities of supervision, etc.

Conclusion

These considerations represent only a schematic view of the multiple and varied ideas expressed in the II Hague Workshop. By offering the opportunity to the representatives of a psychotherapeutic technique to demonstrate their experiences and by obliging them to clarify their ideas and assumptions, these workshops contribute in an important way to the maturation process of this therapy form.

References

Davanloo, H.: Basic principles and techniques in short-term dynamic psychotherapy (Medical & Scientific Books, New York 1978).

Frankel, F.H.: Short-term psychotherapy and hypnosis. Communication at II Hague Workshop on Short-Term Dynamic Psychotherapy, 1980.

Gilliéron, E.: New aspects of short-term dynamic psychotherapy. Communication at II Hague Workshop on Short-Term Dynamic Psychotherapy, 1980.
Heiberg, A.N.: Training in short-term dynamic psychotherapy. Communication at II Hague Workshop on Short-Term Dynamic Psychotherapy, 1980.
Leibovich, M.A.: Short-term psychotherapy and borderline personality. Communication at II Hague Workshop on Short-Term Dynamic Psychotherapy, 1980.
Malan, D.H.: A study of brief psychotherapy (Tavistock, London 1963).
Malan, D.H.: Toward the validation of dynamic psychotherapy (Plenum Press, New York 1976a).
Malan, D.H.: The frontier of brief psychotherapy (Plenum Press, New York 1976b).
Meyer, A.E.: Content analysis of focus formulations, relations to outcome and other variables. Communication at II Hague Workshop on Short-Term Dynamic Psychotherapy, 1980.
Sifneos, P.E.: Short-term dynamic psychotherapy (Plenum Press, New York 1979).

Roland Pierloot, MD, Universitair Psychiatrisch Centrum 'St. Jozef',
Leuvensesteenweg 517, B–3070 Kortenberg (Belgium)

Book Review

Walter Spiel (ed.)

Die Psychologie der 20. Jahrhunderts, Vol. 11/12:

Konsequenzen für die Pädagogik
Kindler, München 1980
vol. 11: 954 pp.; DM 220.–. ISBN 3-463-24011-4
vol. 12: 923 pp.; DM 220.–. ISBN 3-463-24012-2

Dr. *Walter Spiel,* Professor of Neuropsychiatry concerning childhood and adolescence, and Chairman, University of Vienna, is the editor of these two volumes with regard to the Kindler encyclopedia entitled 'Psychology of the twentieth century'. The main title of these two volumes is 'Consequences concerning pedagogy'. With regard to the 89 authors, 29 are doctors and 23 psychologists. Initially, on the outside cover, *Spiel* signalizes his very modern and clearly convincing concept on the basis of four pictures which concern the internationally well-known researchers: *August Aichhorn* and *Hans Zulliger* (vol. XI) as well as *Anna Freud* and *René Spitz* (vol. XII). *Aichhorn* from Austria and *Zulliger* from Switzerland, in both cases pedagogues, have interceded for the psychoanalytically orientated pedagogy by which they mastered the problems with regard to school practice and home care. By *Anna Freud,* the daughter of *Sigmund Freud,* and *René Spitz,* in both cases psychoanalysts, decisive empirical findings with regard to the high psychodynamical relevance concerning the mother-child relationship were elaborated. The great importance of this pedagogic volume also for the doctor is markedly clarified on the basis of the pointed presentation of *Anna Freud's* and *Spitz's* findings which are so unusually important.

The two volumes particularly deal with the problems concerning the maturation – and development – years of the human being. With regard to the consequences for education and therapy, the scientific positions concerning the depth psychologies, the developmental psychology, the biological maturation processes and the social environment are carefully worked out. The inherent normal and pathological psychological phenomena are successfully presented in the two volumes homogenously and didactically. In the doctor's view, the psychologico-medical knowledges with regard to education, therapeutical help, resocialisation and healing pedagogy include an especial relevance. Furthermore, the doctor will emphatically read the chapters concerning the border situations of the human-childlike being.

In contrast to the reviews of the former volumes, the reviewer experienced himself as an interesting learner and not as an expert this time. I was particularly fascinated that the editor was successful in realising a mutual, valid medico-psychologico-pedagogical total concept with regard to the two main subtopics 'Developmental disorders and educational models' (vol. XI) as well as 'Developmental disorders and therapeutical models' (vol. XII). With regard to the content, these two volumes are of unique importance.

H. Freyberger, Hannover

Author Index

Arena, J.G. 64
Armstrong, S. 9

Birgelen, J.H. 217
Blanchard, E.B. 64
Bolz, W. 81, 85, 96, 110, 134, 138, 199
Burzig, G. 134, 138, 199

Deneke, F. 110

Frankl, F.H. 236

Gabel, H. 110
Gilliéron, E. 44, 244

Hartley, D. 9
Hartzuiker, J.A. 218
Heiberg, A.N. 230

Kimm, H.J. 96

Leibovich, M.A. 257
Levitan, H.L. 34

Meyer, A.-E. 81, 85, 96, 110, 134, 138, 199

Østberg, B. 1

Pallmeyer, T.P. 64
Pierloot, R. 55, 265

Rigatelli, M. 22

Sifneos, P.E. 224
Speidel, H. 134
Stuhr, U. 110, 199
Sundsvold, M.Ø. 1

Vaglum, P. 1
Vandereycken, W. 55
Van Londen, J. 221

Yasuna, A. 9

Vol. 35, 1981

Psychotherapy and Psychosomatics

Founded 1953 as 'Acta Psychotherapeutica et Psychosomatica' by E.A.D.E. Carp and B. Stokvis, continued by Th. Spoerri (1964–1974)

Official Organ of the International Federation for Medical Psychotherapy

S. Karger · Basel · München · Paris · London · New York · Sydney

KARGER

S. Karger AG, P.O. Box, CH–4009 Basel (Switzerland)
Printed in Switzerland by Thür AG Offsetdruck, Pratteln

Drug Dosage

The authors and the publisher have exerted every effort to ensure that drug selection and dosage set forth in this text are in accord with current recommendations and practice at the time of publication. However, in view of ongoing research, changes in government regulations, and the constant flow of information relating to drug therapy and drug reactions, the reader is urged to check the package insert for each drug for any change in indications and dosage and for added warnings and precautions. This is particularly important when the recommended agent is a new and/or infrequently employed drug.

Contents Vol. 35, 1981

No. 1

Movements, Lumbar and Temporomandibular Pain and Psychopathology
Sundsvold, M.Ø.; Vaglum, P.; Østberg, B. 1
Brief Psychodynamic Psychotherapy: Interrater Agreement and Reliability of Individually Specified Outcomes
Armstrong, S.; Yasuna, A.; Hartley, D. 9
A Global Psychosomatic Study of 16 Consecutive Patients with Ulcerative Colitis
Rigatelli, M. 22
Patterns of Hostility Revealed in the Fantasies and Dreams of Women with Rheumatoid Arthritis
Levitan, H.L. 34
Influence of the Setting on a Psychotherapeutic Relationship in Analytically Oriented Brief Psychotherapy
Gilliéron, E. 44
Anorexia nervosa in Twins
Vandereycken, W.; Pierloot, R. 55
Psychometric Properties of a Scale to Measure Alexithymia
Blanchard, E.B.; Arena, J.G.; Pallmeyer, T.P. 64

Book Reviews 72
Announcements 76

No. 2-3

The Hamburg Short Psychotherapy Comparison Experiment

Editor: A.-E. Meyer, Hamburg

Foreword and Introduction
Meyer, A.-E.; Bolz, W. 81
The General Setting
Bolz, W.; Meyer, A.-E. 85
The Patient Sample: Overt and Covert Selection Factors and Prognostic Predictions
Kimm, H.J.; Bolz, W.; Meyer, A.-E. 96
Our Focus Formulations: Practicability for Therapy; Content Analyses and Relation to Outcome and Other Variables
Gabel, H.; Deneke, F.; Meyer, A.-E.; Bolz, W.; Stuhr, U. 110
Our Pluridimensional Evaluation System for Short Psychotherapy Outcome
Burzig, G.; Speidel, H.; Bolz, W.; Meyer, A.-E. 134

Outcome Results in Psychological Tests
Stuhr, U.; Meyer, A.-E.; Bolz, W. 138
Outcome Results by Clinical Evaluation Based on the Blind Group Ratings
Meyer, A.-E.; Bolz, W.; Stuhr, U.; Burzig, G. 199

Book Reviews 208

No. 4

II Hague Workshop on Short-Term Dynamic Psychotherapy

Editors: J.A. Hartzuiker and J.H. van Birgelen, Leyenburg

Editorial
In Cauda Venenum
Birgelen, J.H. van 217
STDP, for Better and Worse
Hartzuiker, J.A. 218

Short-Term Psychotherapy, a Major Development for Patients and Psychotherapy
Van Londen, J. 221
Short-Term Dynamic Psychotherapy: Its History, Its Impact and Its Future
Sifneos, P.E. 224
Training in Short-Term Psychotherapy. Research Can Be Superb Clinical Training
Heiberg, A.N. 230
Short-Term Psychotherapy and Hypnosis
Frankl, F.H. 236
Psychoanalysis and Brief Psychotherapy: Some New Considerations on the Psychotherapeutic Process
Gilliéron, E. 244
Short-Term Psychotherapy for the Borderline Personality Disorder
Leibovich, M.A. 257
Short-Term Dynamic Psychotherapy: Progress, Problems, Perspectives
Pierloot, R. 265

Book Review 271
Author Index 272
Contents Vol. 35 .... after 273

Modern Problems of Pharmacopsychiatry, Vol. 14

Series Editors
Th.A. Ban, Nashville, Tenn. P. Pichot, Paris
F.A. Freyhan, Washington, D.C. W. Pöldinger, Wil/St. Gallen

Differential Psychopharmacology of Anxiolytics and Sedatives

Volume Editor
J.-R. Boissier, Romainville
VI + 174 p., 14 fig., 26 tab., 1979
SFr. 54.– / DM 65.– / approx. US $ 32.50
ISBN 3–8055–2777–2

We now recognize that tranquilizing drugs share a fundamental property of being anxiolytic. We also know that sedatives, such as barbiturates, are capable of producing an anxiolytic effect. What remains in question, however, is whether anxiolytic action can be invoked without also inducing sedation.
Papers in this volume explore the differential psychopharmacology of anxiolytics and sedatives in an effort to determine whether their actions can be separated. Clinical, pharmacological, neuropharmacological and behavioral factors are considered in 5 reports authored by internationally recognized experts. Although currently available drugs do not permit a definitive conclusion, research in this volume encourages the possibility that anxiolytic and sedative activities can be dissociated. The volume makes a major contribution to our understanding of the psychopharmacology of tranquilizers. Its information should be particularly useful in the further development of drugs to treat human aggressivity.

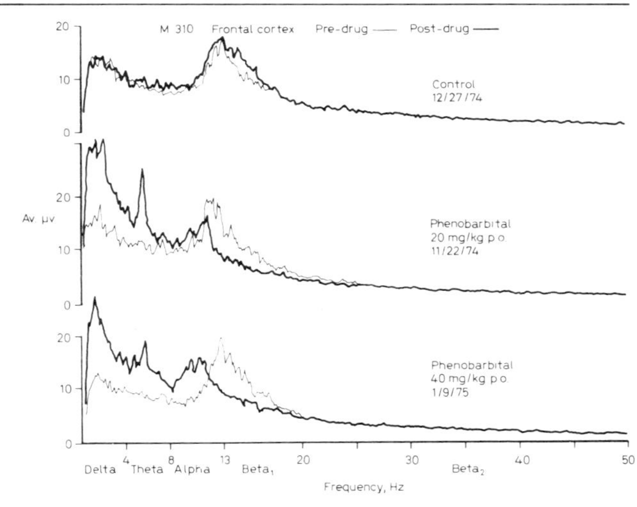

Spectral density analysis of drug effects on ECoG of frontal cortex of squirrel monkey. The spectra show how the electrical energy produced by the brain is distributed over frequency. Each ordinate shows average distribution of peak-to-peak energy µV; the abscissa shows frequency from 0.1–50 Hz. Thin line is predrug, thick line 2 h postdrug. Treatments from top to bottom are control, pheno-at the slow end of the spectrum. (From W. Schallek and W. Schlosser, page 163.)

S. Karger
Basel · München
Paris · London
New York · Sydney

Instructions to Authors

General observations: Only original papers written in English should be sent to:
Dr. Peter E. Sifneos,
Department of Psychiatry,
Harvard Medical School, Beth Israel Hospital,
330 Brookline Avenue,
Boston, MA 02215 (USA).

All manuscripts are subject to editorial review. They should be submitted in triplicate (with three sets of illustrations of which one is an original), typewritten on one side of the paper only and double-spaced with a wide margin. Manuscripts are received with the explicit understanding that they are not under simultaneous consideration by any other publication. It is the author's responsibility to obtain permission to reproduce illustrations, tables, etc. from other publications. Accepted papers become the permanent property of 'Psychotherapy and Psychosomatics' and may not be reproduced by any means, in whole or in part without the written consent of both the author and the publisher.

Arrangement:

Title page: The first page of each paper should carry the title (main title underlined), the authors' names and the name of the institute where the work was done. A short title for use as running head is also to be provided.

Abstract: Each paper must have an abstract of up to 10 lines.

Small type: Paragraphs which can or must be set in smaller type (case histories, test methods, etc.) should be indicated with a 'p' (petit) in the margin on the left-hand side.

Footnotes: They should be avoided. If essential, they appear at the bottom of the respective page and must be numbered consecutively.

Tables and illustrations: Tables (numbered in Roman numerals) and illustrations (numbered in Arabic numerals) should be prepared on separate sheets. They must have a heading resp. a legend, also prepared on a separate sheet. For the reproduction of illustrations, good drawings and original photographs should be submitted; negatives or photocopies cannot be used. If possible, several illustrations should be grouped on one block for reproduction (max. size 113 × 176 mm) or crop marks should be given. On the back of each illustration, its number, the author's name as well as 'top' and 'bottom' have to be indicated. Colored illustrations are reproduced at the authors' expense.

References: The list of references should include only those publications which are cited in the text. They must be arranged alphabetically (citation by name and year) or numbered consecutively (citation by number).

a) Papers published in periodicals: 1. All authors' surnames ('et al.' is not sufficient) with initials of first names; 2. Full title of paper; 3. Journal abbreviation; 4. Volume (in Arabic numerals, underlined and followed by a colon); 5. First and last page; 6. Year of publication in brackets. Example: McIntosh, J.; Hansen, P.; Ziegler, J.; Penny, R.: Defective immune and phagocytic functions in uraemia and renal transplantation. Int. Archs Allergy appl. Immun. 51: 529–540 (1976).

b) Books: 1. Authors' surnames with initials of first names; 2. Full title; 3. In brackets, name and domicile of publishers and year of publication. Example: Pollack, R.S.: Tumor surgery of the head and neck (Karger, Basel 1975).

Full address: The exact postal address complete with postal code of senior author must be given. Should correspondence be handled by someone other, it should be indicated accordingly.

Further details: Authors may consult our leaflet 'Rules for the Preparation of Manuscripts'. This may be obtained free of charge from the Publishers S. Karger AG, P.O. Box, CH–4009 Basel (Switzerland).

Page charges: There is no page charge for papers of 12 printed pages (including tables, illustrations and references) or less. Additional pages or fraction thereof are charged to the authors at SFr. 175.– / US $ 100.00 per page. The allotted size of a paper is equal to approx. 18 manuscript pages (including tables, illustrations and references).

Galley proofs: They will be sent to the first-named author unless otherwise indicated and should be returned with the least possible delay. Alterations made in galley proofs, other than the corrections of printers' errors, will be charged to the author. No page proofs will be supplied.

Reprints: They are available against payment. Order forms with a price list will be sent with the galley proofs. Orders submitted after the issue is printed are subject to considerably higher prices. Allow four weeks from date of publication for delivery of reprints (surface mail; airmail delivery on request and at charge).